The Vince Graham 7 Minute A Day Miracle Body Sculpting Programme

Copyright © Streetwise Publications

First published in Great Britain by

Streetwise Publications
Eden House
Genesis Park
Sheffield Road
Rotherham
S60 1DX

A catalogue record for this book is available from the British Library.

ISBN 09541187-5-8

CONTENTS

FOREWORD

Ever since my early teens I've had a passion for health and fitness. From an early age I craved for the broad shoulders and classic 'V' shaped torso that both men and women admire. I spent many years slaving away in the gym to create such a body. By age 17 I'd left school with lousy exam grades but a reasonable physique.

My parents pressured me to get a job or join the army so that I could "make something of myself", but all I wanted to do was train. Then I had a great idea. I really needed a job (money doesn't grow on trees) and I had that passion for health and fitness so I decided that I would become a gym instructor. It was obvious really. That way I could earn money doing what I enjoy most – training!

I'd found my ideal career and, I enjoyed the job for many years. Then I began to notice something really strange...

99% of gym members didn't seem to make any progress at all. They'd spent £400 a year, or more, on a gym membership, but despite all the effort, looked pretty much the same as the day they'd first walked through the door. They were a bit fitter, but cosmetically there was usually no improvement at all.

At first I assumed the problem was laziness. They just weren't working hard enough. If they put in the effort, they'd get the rewards. But I was wrong.

Because as I was soon to discover, the real reason they had made zero improvement was that they had been misinformed and misled... force-fed a boatload of useless nonsense that was actually pre-venting them from sculpting the body they wanted. And the worst thing of all was that I was one of the people responsible.

I discovered this truth whilst on a business trip to Canada.

About 3 years ago, I was introduced to a friend of a friend on a visit to Ontario. I guessed Vince was in his early fifties, but he had the body of a man 20 years younger, with broad shoulders, mus-cular arms and not a trace of a paunch. He had that classic 'V' shape which both men and women admire...

Being in 'the business' I couldn't resist asking him which gym he used and what sort of equipment he worked out on. Vince smiled broadly, and said that he'd never set foot in a gym in his life, and all the equipment he'd ever used to get in shape was within 6 feet of where we were standing...in his living room!

As a hardened equipment and gym junkie, I just couldn't believe this. I mean, I'd seen hundreds of people slave away in the gym and not get even close to looking as good as Vince. And here he was, telling me that he'd never been to a gym. But there was more...

Because the next thing he told me was that he never worked out for more than 7 minutes a day! Seven minutes! Needless to say, I was intrigued. Over the next hour and a half I became Vince's worst nightmare - quizzing him for every last detail of what he did and how he did it. I was enthralled as he revealed secret after secret of the revolutionary body sculpting system he'd come up with...the little 'twists' and techniques he'd developed to transform himself from a typical overweight couch potato, to a taut, muscular and athletic man of...72 years of age.

That's right...as we spoke, Vince revealed that he would be 73 next birthday!

He told me how he'd worked as an academic all his life, and never really given much thought to his body until he started to approach retirement. He woke up one day, looked in the mirror, saw this old, fat man staring back...and decided to take action.

Where most people would have headed for the gym, Vince headed for the library... that's academics for you...and read every last piece of literature he could find on exercise and body shaping.

At first, it was all pretty confusing, but bit-by-bit the mist cleared, and he started piecing together a system which was radically different to anything being taught in gyms. A system which ordinary people could use to make extra-ordinary progress...and in less time than had previously been thought possible.

That conversation with Vince was like a light coming on in my head. The more I thought about it, the more I realised how much sense it made…and how counterproductive the methods commonly being taught in gyms really were.

Within a few weeks of returning from Canada I'd quit my gym job and since then I've been working as a personal trainer teaching people the Vince Graham 7 Minute A Day Body Sculpting Programme. And now, three years later, I've prepared this programme to share Vince's secrets with you too.

Just one thing before I begin – I'm not a writer, so I hope you'll bear with me. What I'll try to do is communicate the essential information you need as clearly as possible. But don't expect any award winning prose. Hopefully my enthusiasm will overcome any literary shortcomings, and in any event, my guess is that you are reading this in a quest for results – not entertainment.

Everyone who's tried Vince's system has been astonished by the results and I don't expect you to be the exception. I know you're going to achieve massive breakthrough success with this, and envy you that voyage of discovery.

INTRODUCTION

The fact that you're reading this book means that I can safely make a couple of assumptions about you.

It goes without saying that you want to make improvements to the way your body looks, but more than that, you want to do it in the least possible time. That probably means that you're busy. You have a lot going on. You want and need to get results fast. You don't have the time or inclination marathon training sessions...and you don't have the time or inclination to read and de-tangle a mass of information and theory either.

Well the good news is that you don't have to indulge in long and laborious exercise routines, or build an encyclopaedic knowledge of the workings of the human body and exercise theory, to make the sort of improvements that most people can only dream about...

But you do have to do SOMETHING!

And to understand what that something is, and why it works, it's important that you have a basic knowledge of the key muscle groups of the body, what they do, and the triggers that force them to change shape and grow. You also need to familiarise yourself with some pretty unorthodox exercise techniques which simply aren't taught in a regular health club.

For that reason, I'll be starting out by laying some foundations... foundations which will give you a working understanding of how your muscles work, and why the exercise programme we're going to talk about later, is the most efficient and effective for transforming your body from what it is now, to what you want it to be.

I know you'll be keen to get started with the system, but I hope you'll spend a little time studying the next couple of chapters. It's far better to understand exactly why you're doing something, than to do it simply because 'that's what the programme says'.

There's nothing difficult to understand or complicated about any of this, but I know from personal experience that it's information which comes as a genuine revelation to people who have been aimlessly (or misguidedly) slaving away at ineffective and inappropriate exercise routines... routines which give them little chance of success.

I know you're going to enjoy putting Vince's System to work for you, and benefit from it in so many ways. It's going to change the way you look and the way you exercise for as long as you choose to use it.

So let's get started...

CHAPTER ONE
Muscles, Muscles...
And More Muscles!

This is called The Vince Graham 7 Minute A Day BODY SCULPTING programme. It might seem obvious, but I think we need to start by identifying and understanding exactly what we mean (or to be more accurate – what I mean) by a good physique. In other words, what type of body are we trying to sculpt?

The Importance Of Proportion

When I spoke to Vince, he described the perfect physique in terms of achieving the most aesthetically pleasing proportions. Please understand this, because it's important. We're not talking about attaining maximum size...we'll leave that to the bodybuilders. No...we're talking about developing a physique where all parts of the body are in proportion, and where as a result, there's a synergy in which the whole is more impressive and pleasing than the composition of its parts.

I'm beginning to make you sound like an A irfix model, so I think I'd better explain!

What Vince means by proportion, is that it's important to create a 'V' shaped torso, so that when observed head-on, the body appears to be broad at the top (through well developed shoulder and back muscles) before tapering down to a slim waistline. He also stressed that this 'V' shape should be carried through to when the body is viewed from the side as well. This means that the chest muscles should protrude more than the stomach.

In order to remain in proportion, the arms and legs must also be well developed. I must stress here, that all body parts must be trained equally as your body will lose proportion if you have, say, a toned chest but poor leg muscles.

Muscle Is The Key

You can therefore conclude from this that the most important aspect of an aesthetically pleasing body is muscle. Don't panic though! By muscle I don't necessarily mean oversized bodybuilder muscles.

I've lost count of the number of people who've told me that they want to look better, but they don't want to build muscle. Well I've got news for you...the only way you're ever going to improve the way you look is by building your muscles...or at least changing the tone, shape and proportions of them. And the only way you're going to do that is by subjecting them to demands they're not accustomed to.

You know, it really makes me laugh when I see people come into a gym and spend an hour on the running machine and then another half hour on the stationary bike...and then go home. Let me ask you this...do those people have aesthetically pleasing bodies? Do distance runners look good?

If you answered positively, then maybe this isn't the book for you. The fact is that this kind of exercise may be good for your heart and lungs, but it will do little or nothing to make you look better. Why? Because it doesn't put demands on your muscles which will cause them to adapt and change. We'll be going into that in a lot more detail later.

Women in particular, are often fearful of getting involved in exercise programmes designed to impact on muscles. They shouldn't be. The Vince Graham Bodysculpting Programme won't transform your feminine curves into a Desperate Dan like masculine body. In fact many female celebrities use resistance training to keep the body taught and firm and eliminate those 'wobbly bits'. Women are unable to develop muscle in the way that men can because they only have one tenth of the amount of testosterone that men do.

The truth is that most men find it notoriously difficult to build heavy muscle, the exceptions being genetic 'freaks' and those who have found a route via the hypodermic syringe. So women have absolutely nothing to fear on that score.

Resistance Training – What You Need To Know

In our quest to sculpt the perfect body, it 's important to realise why we are doing the exercise we are, and what effect they will have on our bodies in terms of strength and appearance. In this section I'll introduce you to the basic principles of resistance training so that you can understand the benefit of each exercise.

Vince's programme only takes 7 minutes a day, but I'm not going to pretend it's easy. The more you know about the benefits…the more bearable the effort will be for you.

Aside from strengthening, shaping and building the muscles, there is an important additional benefit to resistance training…. it helps to burn fat. Merely by training the muscles, your body will burn excess carbohydrates because this energy is needed when performing such physically demanding exercises.

Also, when the body is stronger with more muscle, you will find that any cardiovascular exercise you do has a greater calorie burning impact because the stronger muscles force your body to burn more calories. Put simply, the more muscle you have, the more fuel it needs to keep going. Just moving a muscular body around during normal day-to-day activities burns more calories than moving a scrawny or fat body around.

The thought that the muscle you've built is silently and effortlessly burning up some of the excess calories you may have consumed, is a very comforting one.

Above, I have noted the two main aesthetic benefits of resistance training – firmer muscles and less fat. However, there are a number of other health related benefits that should not be overlooked.

During intense muscular activity, the heart is required to pump blood to the muscles being worked in order to provide those muscles with energy and nutrients. This in turn strengthens the heart muscle and will also improve circulation.

Another advantage of stronger muscles is that you will become less prone to injury. A stronger muscle will be much more difficult to injure when performing every day tasks. Stronger lower back and abdominal muscles will help to support the spine during lifting and reduce the risk of back injury, which can cause many long-term problems.

Making Muscles Change

So now that we appreciate the value of resistance training and the benefits of making muscles bigger, stronger and more shapely, how specifically, do we go about bringing these changes about. This is simple really.

To make the muscles stronger, we must damage them! This may sound a little strange, but in order for the muscles to change we must damage the muscle fibres. Please note that this is not the same as injuring them.

By exercising a muscle through resistance training, fibres within the muscle are actually damaged. If we then rest the muscle, our bodies will repair the damage and will also make the muscle stronger than it previously was. This is the main principle behind all muscle building programmes – you exercise the muscle and it will grow stronger.

Your muscles are placed under stress to which they are not accustomed. As a result the fibres are broken down to some degree, and subsequently repair themselves. But they do not repair themselves to the way they were before…they adapt to the new demands that have been placed on them, and grow bigger and stronger as a result.

Changing the strength and size of a muscle is deceptively simple!

1. Place it under stress to which it isn't accustomed.
2. Give it time to recover and adapt to the new demands.
3. Repeat!

The mechanics of exactly how to do this in the fastest and most efficient manner are a little more complicated, and that's what you're about to learn in the rest of this book.

The Major Muscle Groups

Here's something strange I used to find in the gym. There were people there who had been happily (well maybe not happily!) sweating away over exercise programmes for years…and when questioned didn't have even the most basic knowledge of human anatomy. They had no real idea what each group of muscles did, or which muscles they were working on with each exercise.

It's almost impossible to maximise the results you're getting if you don't know what you're working on, so with that in mind (and apologies if your knowledge in these matters is more detailed than most) I'm going to give you a basic overview of the major muscle groups of the body…and most importantly…exactly what they do.

Anterior Muscles

Posterior Muscles

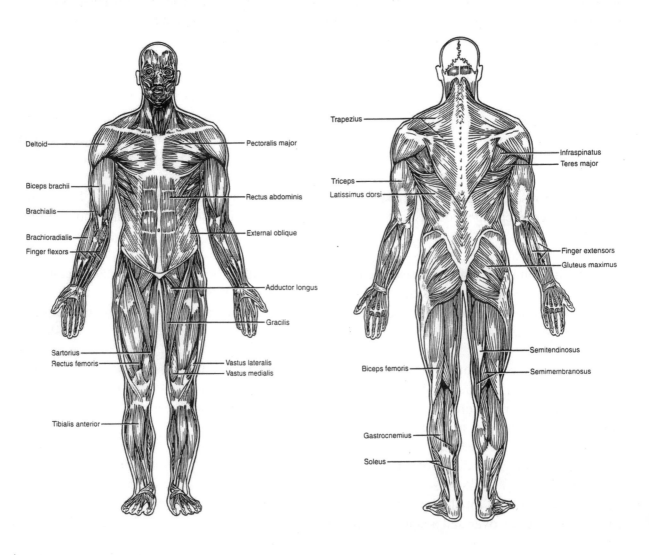

Deltoid

Biceps brachii

Brachialis

Brachioradialis

Finger flexors

Pectoralis major

Rectus abdominis

External oblique

Adductor longus

Gracilis

Sartorius

Rectus femoris

Vastus lateralis

Vastus medialis

Tibialis anterior

Trapezius

Triceps

Latissimus dorsi

Infraspinatus

Teres major

Finger extensors

Gluteus maximus

Semitendinosus

Biceps femoris

Semimembranosus

Gastrocnemius

Soleus

Arms

Yes, I know you know what arms are, but do you know how they're made up, or what they do? If you're asked to 'show your muscles', the biceps muscle in the upper arm is usually the one that you will tense. I don't really know why this is…something to do with Popeye probably…but it's a fact. For women, the firm triceps muscles will help to eliminate sagging flesh on the underside of the arms, referred to in the fitness world as 'bingo wings'!

The arms can be divided into upper arms (between the shoulder and elbow) and the forearms (between the elbow and wrist). The upper arm consists of the biceps (the ones you use for showing off) and the triceps… the muscles at the back of the arm opposite to the biceps.

The biceps is actually two muscles. The word 'biceps' means two heads. The biceps brachii is the peak of the muscle, which sits on top the larger brachialis underneath. These muscles are involved in pulling movements and enable you to bend your arm towards you. Typical exercises for these muscles would involve a curling movement where a weight is lifted from your sides at hip level up towards your chest and shoulders, with the upper arm stationary.

The triceps muscles are the opposite of the biceps in terms of location and function. The triceps are located on the opposite side of your upper arm to the biceps at the back of your arm. As the name suggests, there are three 'heads' to the triceps muscle which when properly developed can greatly improve the definition of the upper arm. The triceps muscles are involved in pushing movements and enable you to straighten your arm and extend your hand away from your body.

The forearms consist of the brachioradials, flexor and extensor muscles. The forearms are used mostly in the movement of the hand and wrist and are important for grip. Exercises do exist that concentrate solely on muscles in the forearms but it is my opinion that it is unnecessary to perform them as the forearms are involved as secondary muscles in exercises that involve the upper arms so they will be worked enough anyway. More about that later.

Shoulders

Broad shoulders are essential to a well-developed physique. They help to accentuate the 'V' shaped torso and also provide an optical illusion, by giving the impression that your waistline is smaller than it really is.

Strong shoulders are also beneficial to every other muscle group in the upper body in that they are involved in exercises that work the chest, back and arm muscles as well. With stronger shoulders, you will be able to put more effort into the workouts for your other body parts.

There are two main muscle groups in the shoulders - the deltoid muscles and the trapezius muscles. There are two deltoid muscles, one in each of your shoulders extending from your collarbone to your upper arms. The deltoids, like the triceps, have three 'heads' the anterior, lateral and posterior deltoids meaning front, side and back 'heads' of the muscle. These muscles are involved in raising and rotating the arms. Typical exercises focusing on these muscles include lifting weights above the head and raising weights up to the front, sides and rear of the body.

The trapezius muscles are used to raise your shoulders and rotate your shoulder blades. They are the muscles that slope up from your deltoid muscles to the sides of the neck. They are involved in many of the back exercises, but can also be trained individually.

Chest

A strong chest is crucial when sculpting the perfect body. In men, a well-developed chest conveys strength and power and is a source of physical attractiveness. In a study carried out at Newcastle University, 30 female students were asked to rank 50 colour photos of male torsos. The men with the best chest-to-waist ratio were ranked the most attractive. The researches concluded that the 'V' shaped torso is very much a desired characteristic, with broad chest and shoulders and a narrow waist.

Developing the chest muscles is also important for women, as developing the muscles will help to support the breasts.

The chest is involved in pushing movements such as press-ups or if your car fails to start and requires some human-power to get it going. Your chest muscles are called the pectorals (or pecs) and there are two muscles on each side of the chest. The pectoralis major is the larger of the two, and is a large piece of muscle spanning the top of the chest. Below it is the pectoralis minor.

You may have guessed by now that because the muscle groups are composed of different parts (e.g. pectoralis major and minor) that each part of the muscle may be developed by different tweaks to each exercise. The 7-minute workout ensures that no muscle, major or minor, is neglected.

Abdominal Muscles

The abdominal muscles are a vital muscle group to develop because strong abdominals promote good posture, support the back, and provide protection for the internal organs. They also provide a core to the body. If the core is strong, you will be able to develop more power when performing other exercises.

I really don't think I need to tell you that a flat stomach is usually appealing to the opposite sex. Well-developed abdominal muscles will help a man to achieve that 'six-pack' look, or a woman to obtain a trim and toned waistline.

However, here's the bad news. We've all got 'abs' to some extent but nobody will ever see them if they are covered by three inches of fat. To really see these highly desirable muscles will require some work. Not only must we train the muscles well (and I will show the one exercise that works better than the rest) but we must also lose the fat that covers those muscles through a sensible eating regime and cardiovascular exercise. I will come back to these points in later chapters.

The abdominals are actually comprised of three different muscle groups. The most notable are the rectus abdominis, which are those 'six-pack' muscles that run from the sternum to the navel. Hidden behind these muscles is the transversus abdominis that form the 'core' I mentioned earlier. These muscles, although they cannot be seen are important for posture and support.

The third and final group of muscles in your mid-section are known as the obliques and can be found extending up and down your sides. If you cannot find them, they may be hiding beneath what are commonly known as 'love-handles'. Don't worry if they are, we will soon whip you into shape!

Back

Many people pay little attention to their back muscles. This is simply because they are difficult to see. However, in Vince's opinion (and I agree with him) they are equally if not more important than the chest muscles. You see, the back muscles are the key to developing that 'V' shape I've been talking about.

You should be able to see your back muscles from the front when you raise your arms. Even more than the shoulders or chest, well-developed back muscles have an incredible ability to visually reduce the size of the waistline. In-fact, the largest muscles in the entire upper body are in your back. These are known as the latissimus dorsi muscles and extend from behind each armpit to the middle of your lower back. They are two (one on each side of the spine) large triangular slabs of muscle that actually add more size to your chest measurement than your pectoral muscles do. When they are trained, they add width to your upper torso.

The other major back muscles are known as the rhomboideus or rhomboid muscles and are found between the shoulder blades and the spine. These muscles are much smaller than the latissimus dorsi muscles but add thickness to the upper back.

The main muscles in the lower back are know as the erector spinae and are the counterparts to the abdominal muscles. They work together with the 'abs' to support the back during lifting, twisting, and flexing movements. They add little to appearance but are crucial in avoiding back problems in later life.

Legs

The legs make up almost half of your body and yet during my time spent as a gym instructor I would see many people train for an hour and not even bother training their leg muscles at all. The reason Vince looks so great is down to proportionality, remember? If you have a great muscular upper body but legs like pipe cleaners, you just won't look right. You need to train the leg muscles at least once a week or face having an imbalanced physique.

It goes without saying that the leg muscles are very important for women, and to be fair, in my experience, they seem to neglect them far less than men. Something to do with wearing skirts and dresses I'd imagine. Wonder if Scotsmen neglect leg training as much as Englishmen?

The thighs are made up of two very large muscle groups: the quadriceps and the hamstrings. The quadriceps are located at the front of the thighs and as the name suggests, they have four 'heads'. The quadriceps are involved in movements that require you to extend your knee. If you have ever been told to lift with your legs and not your back, it is the quadriceps' that are being used. Strong quadriceps will also help reduce the risk of injury to the knees.

The hamstrings are located at the back of the leg between the knee and the buttocks. The hamstrings are comprised of three 'heads' and thus are not as strong as the quadriceps. They are involved in movements that bend the knee such as if you raise your heel up towards your buttocks. Many exercises actually train the quadriceps and the hamstrings at the same time so little attention needs to be paid in exercising the muscles separately.

The only leg muscle, which must be exercised separately, is the calf muscle. This is a much neglected muscle but can actually be trained quite easily. Many men who consider themselves as having 'skinny legs' really only have skinny calves. The calves are located on the back of the lower leg and consist of two muscles the gastrocnemius and the soleus. The gastroncnemius is located on top of the soleus muscle and when properly developed forms a diamond shape.

Buttocks

Believe it or not, the muscles in your buttocks are larger than any other muscle group in your entire body. Each dare I say it – cheek, contains three muscles. The gluteus maximus being the largest. Beneath this muscle are the smaller gluteus medius and gluteus minimus.

The 'glutes' as they are called in gym speak are not a muscle group to... errm... turn the other cheek on. In numerous studies, le derriere always turns out to be the physical feature voted to be most attractive by both men and women. The bottom line is this: we must tone the tush to maintain an overall attractive appearance.

The good news however is this: we don't have to actually devote a single day to train the backside. Many leg exercises actually include the 'glutes' as a secondary or even primary muscle group. We can therefore incorporate the leg and buttocks workout into one training session

Having now looked at each of the major muscle groups, you should now have a good understanding of what each one does, what it looks like, and the type of movements, which will be involved in developing it. Vince has carefully developed the programme as a result of many years of research and experimentation, to enable us to work each of these muscles in the best possible way and in the least amount of time.

In the next chapter I would like to tell you why you, and many people like you, have being wasting your money in gyms and health clubs and have nothing to show for it.

CHAPTER TWO
Vince v The Rest

Why Have Previous Efforts Failed?

After I met Vince, I realised that the health clubs and gyms have been teaching people out of date methods and techniques that fail to produce solid, measurable results. It also dawned on me that for the first seven years of my career I had been guilty of the same thing. This was not intentional. I was doing my best...what I thought was right... but I'd been misinformed, just as everybody else has. The only reason that I had experienced any personal results whatsoever was down to a combination of favourable genetics and hours and hours spent slaving away at the gym.

The reason that few people experience measurable improvements is a direct result of the profit driven nature of the fitness industry. That's not a criticism...everybody has to make a profit...but it does have some negative consequences.

Devices And Gadgets

The men behind the scenes spend a great deal of time thinking up new nick-nacks and gadgets to sell to as many 'mugs' as possible. Make no mistake...the starting point for these gadgets is not a prototype which is proven to work...it's an idea which looks like it will sell!

The exercise equipment hawkers sell tens of thousands of ineffective devices, such as silly sit up devices and bits of plastic that you stick on your body to make you twitch in your armchair at home – what a joke! I have never met a single person who has sat on their backside with one of those electrical impulse gadgets and made even the slightest improvement.

With this system, everything you will need is in your home right now. In a later chapter I will show you how to construct your own DIY home gym.

Gyms And Health Clubs

Most people make little improvements at the gym, because they haven't been shown the most effective way to train. When you visit a gym, an instructor is likely to put you on a machine to train a particular muscle for a minute or two and then move you onto another machine to train a different muscle. And then on to another machine and another until you've been in the gym for an hour...and you haven't even trained a single muscle properly!

The reason the instructors are keen to move you from machine to machine is that they want to move people around the gym as quickly as possible so that queuing for machines is minimised. However, the downside to this is that you only spend a couple of minutes training one muscle group and then you forget about it and train another. This will never produce results, as a muscle group requires more than two minutes of work per session to respond to the training.

A typical routine (actually this is better than most) would look something like this: (Don't worry if you don't understand any of these exercises…this section is really for those who've tried and failed.)

Chest: Bench press machine
Back: Pull-down machine
Shoulders: Shoulder-press machine
Biceps: Dumbbell curls
Triceps: Dumbbell kickbacks
Legs: Seated leg-press machine
Abdominals: Sit-ups

Typically you would be required to perform each exercise for ten repetitions, you may then rest for a minute and perform another ten repetitions until you have completed two or three 'sets' of ten repetitions. The instructors would then recommend that you perform this routine three times a week (maybe on Monday, Wednesday and Friday).

Performing the exercises in such a way is pointless as your body does not understand such things as 'sets' and 'repetitions'. All that your body understands is the amount of work it has done in a given time. If you rest for a minute between sets in the above workout, you will waste around 15 minutes of your workout sat down doing nothing.

There are three main reasons that such workouts are ineffective:

1. Very little time is spent exercising each muscle group, because the instructor has tried to cram the whole body into one workout. As a result, none of the muscles have been trained intensively enough for the workout to be effective.

2. Workouts lack variety. In the first chapter, I explained how the muscle fibres respond to intense activity because, as a result of training the fibres are damaged and then grow back stronger. In order for this process to continue in the long term, you must surprise the muscles. If you stick to the same programme of three 'sets' of ten 'repetitions' and perform the same exercises week-in week-out, the muscles will become used to this stimulus and will no longer respond.

3. The final step on the gym-members' road to failure is that the same muscles are constantly put under stress. You are training the same part of the same muscle group three times a week. Admittedly only for a couple of minutes but the muscles require a more significant rest period between training sessions. It is counter-productive to train the same muscle on two consecutive training days because the muscle actually firms up and grows when it is resting, not when it is working. If a muscle is trained too often, it will simply break down and become weaker or at the very least, remain the same. We learned in the first chapter that the muscle actually grows and becomes stronger when we rest, not when we train. The above routine would only succeed in repetitively damaging the muscles.

Why Will The Vince Graham 7-Minute A Day Body Sculpting Programme Succeed?

The Vince Graham programme addresses all of the problems associated with a regular resistance routine in that it incorporates a trio of core principles…

1. Intensity and focus
2. Variety
3. Adequate Rest

As a solution to the first problem encountered with the typical workout, the Vince Graham programme embraces the fact that it is much more effective to spend the whole session working one muscle group in different ways, than it is to train the whole body in one session. Also, because the body does not understand the concept of 'sets and reps', Vince prefers to measure performance based on the amount of work completed in a given time period. This not only reduces wasted rest periods but it helps with motivation by enabling you to set yourself goals.

The second problem encountered was the lack of variety, which results in the body becoming accustomed to the workout and then failing to respond. The Vince Graham programme includes a comprehensive range of exercises, which can be performed at home to add variety to the workout. The system also includes a number of off-the-wall techniques to really shock the body and maintain the ideal changing environment for sculpting the perfect body.

The typical approach can also be criticised on the grounds that it allows little time between workouts for rest and muscle growth. Vince recommends that you train each muscle group only once per week. This allows each muscle exactly one week to rest and grow stronger. By training in this way, the muscles will grow stronger, firmer and larger much more quickly. You will begin to sculpt your body into the perfect physique.

By dedicating a day for training just one muscle group, for example training the chest on Monday, you can spend more time training that specific area, but less time training altogether. This is because you don't need to spend time training the other muscles on Monday. This saves time and effort that would otherwise be used counter-productively.

Core Techniques That Underpin The Vince Graham System

The Vince Graham system utilises a number of principles for body sculpting that have been adapted from the workouts of professional bodybuilders. The fact is that we are aiming to make the most impact on our bodies in the shortest possible time. Bodybuilders are the masters of this.

Now that doesn't mean that we all end up looking like bodybuilders – far from it. But by adopting and adapting the techniques they use, we can get the results and outcomes we're striving for, as quickly as possible.

These techniques have been time proven by research and by professional athletes over a number of years, but are rarely seen in health clubs and gyms. Gym instructors simply don't possess the knowledge to utilise such methods.

I'd now like to spend a little time explaining the key principles that underpin Vince's system. These techniques are what make the system different. They are what make the system so effective. They are the basis of the road by which you are to arrive at your ultimate aesthetic destination.

Continuous Tension

Unlike some of the other techniques that I'm going to talk about, (which will be utilised occasionally to add variety), continuous tension will be incorporated into every workout.

Continuous tension is a key principle in the Vince Graham system because it ensures what is known as a 'peak contraction' within the muscles. When a muscle is contracted, the muscle fibres shorten, making the muscle firm and tense. The term 'peak contraction' refers to the point where all the muscle fibres are engaged in the contraction. This is a very important, and often neglected principle that will dramatically accelerate the results you are striving to achieve.

In order to ensure a 'peak contraction', we must perform as many repetitions as possible under conditions of continuous tension. Continuous tension is achieved by eliminating any resting points during the movement of the exercise. The resting points that I am referring to are any points during the exercise where the muscles are relaxed.

As most people are familiar with the press-up exercise, I'll use the press-up as an example to demonstrate my point...

When performing the press-up, you will start with your hands and toes in contact with the floor. Your back and legs should form a straight line from your feet to your head. Before you commence the movement, your arms will be straight with your elbows locked out. While the elbows are locked-out, the pectoral muscles are not under tension as your weight is supported by the bones in your arm and not by any muscles.

To perform one repetition, you will bend your arms at the elbows and lower your torso down towards the floor. You will then push with your arms to raise your body back up again. To maintain 'continuous tension' in the muscles, when you raise your body back up again you MUST NOT straighten your arms and lock the elbows. By keeping them slightly bent before performing another repetition, the rest period at the top of the movement will be eliminated and you will see better results.

It should be your goal to perform as many repetitions as possible under continuous tension. If you feel you cannot perform another repetition under continuous tension it is acceptable to pause with the elbows locked out before performing more repetitions.

Continuous tension is a powerful technique that can be used with a wide variety of exercises. It ensures that the relevant muscles are kept under constant stress throughout a 'set' of an exercise, and the effectiveness of that exercise is multiplied as a result.

Once we get on to the workout section of the book, I'll be explaining exactly how you can use constant tension to enhance exercises for all your body parts

Supersets

Conventional resistance training employs 'straight sets' as its core principle. A straight set is performed by doing a series of repetitions of a movement... usually somewhere between 8 and 12... then stopping to rest for a minute or so before carrying out a further set.

A superset is an advanced training technique in which you perform two or more exercises in a row, with virtually no rest in between them. Supersets are an excellent technique for muscular development, especially if you are short of time. Supersets are not, the most effective technique for building huge muscles though. Let me explain why...

When you perform multiple exercises, with no rest in between, the weight you're able to use will be limited by the fatigue you're experiencing from the previous exercise. Because supersets don't allow you to use maximal resistance, they are not well-suited to building size.

Supersets are definitely a 'shaping technique'. That's why we are using them. We don't want to look like the Incredible Hulk, we merely want to firm and shape the muscles to give optimal proportions and aesthetic appearance.

Okay, so you now you know what a superset is. The question is; why should you bother using them? There are two primary advantages of superset training over conventional straight set training:

1. Supersets save time.

2. Supersets increase intensity. Vince stresses that the key to the 7-minute workout is intensity. Supersets allow us to maximise the amount of work that we can achieve in 7 minutes.

Supersets In Practice

Super-setting involves combining two or more exercises for the same muscle group... an isolation exercise first, followed by a basic, compound movement. Here's how it works...

There are two main types of exercise...compound and isolation.

Exercises that are intended to train a particular muscle, but also train other muscles, as secondary muscles, are known as compound exercises. A good example of a compound exercise is the press-up. A press-up is primarily an exercise for the pectoral muscles in the chest, but when performing a press-up, the triceps in the back of the arms and deltoids in the shoulders are also worked.

Other movements are referred to as isolation exercises (or concentration exercises). These are exercises that focus entirely on one muscle and do not involve any other muscles as secondary muscles. A common example is the fly, which is an exercise that focuses entirely on the pectoral muscles, in the chest. We'll be learning exactly how to perform that exercise once we get on to the workout.

Now – when you perform a superset, the normal sequence is to perform an isolation exercise, followed immediately by a compound one for the same muscle group. This is to take advantage of a principle called pre-exhaustion.

An example would be super-setting flys with press-ups. So you would perform a set of flys (isolation exercise for the chest) immediately followed by a set of press-ups (compound exercise for the chest). A pre-exhaust superset is performed by choosing two exercises for the same muscle group, and then performing the isolation and compound movements in rapid succession.

The principle of 'pre-exhaustion' utilises isolation and compound exercises to increase the intensity of a workout, and the results you get from it.

In a 'traditional' workout, if you were to perform a set of press-ups (which works the chest but also the triceps) until the point of failure, it would be the triceps, rather than the pectorals that would tire first. They are the smaller and weaker muscles involved in the movement. So, when you are too tired to perform another press-up, your triceps have been worked to the maximum, but your pectorals (which you are trying to work on) haven't even broken sweat.

In order to increase the effectiveness of the press-up as a pectoral exercise then, you can partially tire (pre-exhaust) the pectorals before performing the press-up. Performing an isolation exercise first, such as flys, can achieve this.

Listed below are some examples of exercises that work well together. The first exercises (1) are isolation exercises, the second exercises (2) are compound exercises:

Chest: (1) Flys / (2) Press-ups

Back: (1) Pullovers / (2) Chins

Shoulders: (1) Side Lateral Raises / (2) Shoulder Press

Biceps:(1) Concentration Curls / (2) Curl Grip Chins

Triceps: (1) Triceps French Press / (2) Close Grip Press-ups

Don't worry if you are unfamiliar with these exercises, as we will focus on the different exercises in later chapters. It is important however to make sure you understand the concept of supersets, as they are a central principle of the Vince Graham System.

Super-Slow Movements

I've already discussed the benefits of constant change. In an ideal situation, no one workout would be the same as another, so the Vince Graham system strives to make each workout as varied as possible.

The routine can be altered by performing different exercises, but also through performing the same exercise in different ways. A good example of this would be to perform the exercises at varied speeds. By occasionally performing super slow movements in a workout, the muscle group involved in the exercise is shocked by a change in the pace of movement. This is a highly effective way to produce the results that we are looking for.

The 'super-slow' method can be applied to any exercise but in this instance I will again use the press-up as an example.

Most people are familiar with the press-up. It's an exercise used primarily to tone the chest muscles but also works the triceps and the front deltoid muscles. Typically a normal press-up can be performed in one or two seconds. If a person can perform 25 press-ups, I would consider them to have a good level of fitness. A super-slow press up is much more difficult. It should last around ten seconds in duration (five seconds to lower the body to the floor, five seconds to return to the starting position). In 'super-slow', I would consider only ten repetitions to be good. Because of the increased level of difficulty, the muscles will respond well after much fewer repetitions.

Explosive Power

There are two portions to every exercise – a positive portion and a negative portion. The positive portion is the part of the exercise where you actually lift the weight. For example in a press-up this is the portion where you push your body up from the floor. The part of the exercise where your body is lowered to the floor is the negative portion.

This is the same for all exercises. In a sit up, for example, the positive portion is where you raise your chest towards your knees and the negative portion is the part where you lower your torso back down to the floor.

Another way to add variety to our workouts is to perform some exercises with explosive power. This is where you exert more power and energy than is necessary to the positive portion of the exercise. The negative portion should be performed with normal speed and power. By using explosive power, you develop more strength in the muscles. More strength means that you will be able to put more energy into each workout.

An example of an exercise that utilises explosive power is the 'clap press-up' In this exercise, you exert enough power to the positive portion of the exercise that you are able to remove your hands from the floor and 'clap' them. I must apologise for the repetitive use of the press-up as an example, however, it is the one exercise that almost everybody is familiar with.

When we begin the workout in later chapters, I will introduce you to a wide variety of exercises for each body part. Until then, I hope you'll bear with me.

Negatives

Negatives, as you may have guessed already, emphasise the negative portion of the exercise by performing it more slowly. The positive portion is performed at normal speed and the negative portion is performed at a third of normal speed. The negative portion should not be performed as slowly as super-slow but should be performed very smoothly and under control. We will use negatives in our workouts from time to time to surprise the muscles and add more variety.

CHAPTER THREE
Preparing For Success

In the previous chapters we have already learned a great deal about the human body, and some the weapons in our arsenal that will help us to turn it into the toned, muscular machine we want it to be. As we progress into chapter three, we are almost ready to start working out.

Sculpting the perfect body is not an easy process (if it were we would all be walking round looking like Brad Pitt and Jennifer Aniston). But most of us would agree that it's worth the effort... particularly when we've honed that effort down to 7 minutes a day of hard-boiled, not a second wasted, action.

This chapter will help prepare you both physically and mentally for the battle ahead.

Mind and Body

Before we get down to any physical activity, I want you to understand the importance of the connection between the mind and body.

If you are reading this then your mind has already played an important part in developing your body. It has given you motivation. Your mind has already motivated you to initially buy this book, but subsequently it has motivated you to read the previous two chapters. It is the mind that will also provide you with the self-motivation to train and improve the body. In reality, all motivation is self-motivation. There is no other kind.

The mind is an incredible and powerful organ that you must learn to control and master. When you can control the mind, you can channel its powers to help you achieve anything. And I mean anything. By using this positive power you can achieve success in all areas of life, not just your health and appearance. You can use this power to earn yourself riches, improve your relationships or overcome any challenge that life throws at you.

In order to succeed in sculpting the perfect body it is essential to stay positive and motivated. You must constantly set yourself goals and challenges and when you surpass these goals, you must set more goals. The phrases "I can't" or "I'll do it tomorrow" should not even come in to your mind.

It's important to be crystal clear about exactly what you want to get out of this programme. Why did you buy this book? Perhaps you looked at yourself in the mirror one morning and were unsatisfied by your appearance? Perhaps you are happy with the way you look and just want to be fitter or stronger? Perhaps you want to just firm up certain areas of the body, or maybe you want to add two inches to your biceps measurement.

Whatever the reason, you must focus on this goal, get a clear picture in your mind of your ideal body and work steadily towards it... I cannot do the work for you, and nor can anyone else. I can merely inform you of the best way to go about it. I can teach you the methods that work so you don't waste time on the ones that don't.

Consulting Your Doctor

The Vince Graham system is designed in such a way and with such a variety of exercises that men and women of all ages should be able to gain benefits from performing the exercises. However, it is advisable to visit your GP for a physical examination before any kind of exercise programme is started if you answer "yes" to one or more of the following questions:

- Are you over the age of 45?
- Do you smoke?
- Has anyone in your family suffered a heart attack before the age of 60?
- Has your blood pressure been measured at higher than 140 over 90?
- Is your cholesterol greater than 240?
- Are you physically inactive (less than three sessions of exercise per week for thirty minutes per session)?
- Are you more than 20 pounds overweight?

If you answered "yes" to more than one of the above questions your doctor will probably urge you to exercise but it is advisable to make sure first.

Eating

Fuel is needed to complete any workout, even if it's one lasting no more than 7 minutes. And now I'm going to say something, which you might find rather confusing. You should never work out on an empty stomach…or a full one! I think I'd better explain.

It's best not to exercise on an empty stomach because your body needs energy to perform the exercises. If you train first thing in the morning for example, there is a chance that you may feel light headed, dizzy or even faint because when you sleep, you are effectively fasting. When you wake up, you have very few carbohydrates left in your body to burn for energy.

If, however, you eat a great deal prior to your training session, you are likely to feel nauseous. Following the consumption of food, blood is required in and around the stomach in order to digest the food properly. If you train immediately after a large meal, the blood will go to the muscles rather than to the stomach, meaning your food will be poorly digested.

The solution to this apparent dilemma? I would recommend a light meal or snack half an hour prior to a workout.

Many studies have shown that it is far better to eat five or six small meals per day rather than three large meals. The reason for this is that your body has a constant, moderate supply of energy rather than having a peak in energy at certain times followed by an energy crash.

Also, by having frequent small meals, you will be less tempted to snack on junk food such as sweets and crisps.

Another bonus associated with the frequent meal principle is that you will never be too full to train. In addition to this, frequent meals will help to keep the metabolism high so that your body will burn fat more easily. Every time you eat, your metabolism (the rate at which you burn calories) is temporarily raised. The more often you eat, the more often it's raised.

When I spoke to Vince, he made very clear that he didn't believe in diets, and I'm in full agreement with him on that. Diets never work. By dieting you may be able to lose a few pounds in the first few weeks but this loss will slow down as your metabolism readjusts to lower calorific intake. When you go back to eating normally again, your slower metabolism will result in you putting those pounds back on again.

Rather than dieting, I would suggest simply adopting a sensible balanced diet. In my experience, the worst foods to eat are those containing simple, refined sugars. Basically it's the sweets that make you fat. Your body will use nutrients for energy depending on the complexity of the molecules. Protein is very complex and thus is rarely used for energy. Then come fats, which are moderately complex. Fats will be burned for energy if the carbohydrates are used first. Carbohydrates are the simplest nutrient and thus are the main energy source for our bodies. Sweet foods contain simple carbohydrates, which are easily digested. When they are digested quickly, the body is hit with large quantities of energy that it cannot use. Fats are therefore not needed for energy and are stored. This makes us fat.

If we consume more complex carbohydrates such as those found in oats, muesli, brown bread, brown rice and so on, they take longer to digest, providing a more steady, sustained release of energy. Thus, when larger quantities of energy are required, our bodies will use the complex carbohydrates as well as some fat. The fat is not put into storage and we will remain slim.

A well balanced diet is therefore high in protein (to keep our muscles toned), low in fat (so that this fat cannot be stored), and contains moderate amounts of complex carbohydrates to provide sustained energy release.

The body requires some good fats such as those found in olive oil and flaxseed oil to lubricate the joints and to act as a transport mechanism for vitamins and minerals. It goes without saying that bad fats are to be found in chips, crisps and bacon butties. Sorry folks, I'm afraid you'll have to stop eating junk in order to avoid looking like it. The general rule is this – if it tastes bland and boring it is okay to eat!

In Chapter 11, I'll be looking at nutrition in more detail, and laying the foundations for a lifestyle change which you can easily live with.

Drinking

I'm afraid that this section holds even more bad news. In addition to reducing the amount of fats and sugars you consume, you will also have to reduce the amount of alcohol and caffeine in your diet. Alcohol is a real physique spoiler. Not only does it pack on the calories but it also acts as a diuretic meaning that it dehydrates you. Caffeine also does this.

Water is the best thing that you can possibly drink. You should drink plenty of water to keep your body hydrated. Aim for three litres a day. Our bodies are made up of almost two-thirds water and we need plenty to ensure our skin remains clear and our muscles full and firm. Drinking more water will also be effective in flushing out toxins from your body.

Breathing

Yes I know you know how to breathe, but this is a little bit different. When performing exercises, it is important that you know how to breathe correctly.

It is important to exhale (breathe out) when exerting most effort (during the positive portion of the exercise) and breathe in (inhale) when exerting least effort (negative portion of the exercise). This allows you to generate the most power to perform the movement. That's why javelin throwers always scream at the moment they throw the javelin (screaming is an effective way to exhale). If attempting this, try not to wake the neighbours!

The Structure Of The 7 Minute Workout

We've already discussed the fact that it is more beneficial to train one body part on one day and then rest that muscle group for a week. The 7 minute workout therefore allocates a muscle group to each day of the week with the exception of Sunday which you will be glad to know is a day of rest where we do not train. The allocation of muscle group to days is as follows:

*   Monday: Chest
*   Tuesday: Back
*   Wednesday: Shoulders
*   Thursday: Legs
*   Friday: Arms
*   Saturday: Abdominals
*   Sunday: Rest

It's important that you only train a muscle group on its allocated day and that you do not try to rearrange the programme in any way as Vince's research shows training the muscles in this order to be most effective.

Here's why…

When you train the chest muscles, the shoulders and triceps muscles are used slightly as secondary muscles. And when we train the shoulders, the chest and triceps muscles are used as secondary muscles.

We therefore must leave a day between training the chest, shoulders and triceps to avoid over training the secondary muscles.

The same is true of the back muscles. When we exercise the back muscles, the biceps are used as secondary muscles and therefore we must leave at least one day between training the back and biceps. For this reason, the arms workout (biceps and triceps) is on a Friday, isolated between abdominals (Saturday) and legs (Thursday).

By structuring the workout in this way, we are ensuring that all the muscles are optimally rested. Some people suggest that you should not train on two consecutive days. This is incorrect. You just should not train the same muscle groups on two consecutive days. This workout enables the optimum amount of training and rest period for each muscle group.

Performing The Exercises

When following the instructions of the Vince Graham 7 Minute A Day Body Sculpting Programme, you will be asked to perform exercises for a given amount of time rather than a number of sets or repetitions. If you are asked to perform an exercise for a duration of two minutes, you are not expected to exercise for two minutes without rest. You can rest as many times as you like so long as you perform two minutes' worth of activity. For example, you may exercise for one minute and then rest. You might then resume the exercise for another thirty seconds and then rest before completing the final thirty seconds.

Although I did say you can rest as many times as you want, you will make better improvements if you minimise the amount, frequency and duration of rest periods. Your goal should be to perform your seven-minute workout with as few rests as possible. The ultimate level of fitness that we wish to attain is a point where like Vince we can perform seven minutes of activity in seven minutes. This means no rests at all.

Don't worry if you have to take frequent rests at first. The more practice you get, the stronger and fitter you will become.

Constructing Your DIY Home Gym

One of the objectives of the Vince Graham 7 Minute A Day Body Sculpting Programme is to prevent you from wasting precious time and money on various gadgets and nick-nacks that just don't work. We've all seen the amusing advertisements on dubious satellite TV shopping channels for products that will transform you from a Rik Waller body double into a perfectly toned, six-pack sporting hunk in under four weeks! Yeah right!

While the marketers try their very best to make products sound appealing to us by emphasising wild claims, little effort actually goes into producing a product that works. Good examples are the various pieces of equipment that are supposedly made to carve out those abdominal muscles. You know, the things made of metal tubing that you hold onto while performing sit-ups and crunches. These have actually been scientifically proven not to be any more effective than a regular sit up. And, as Vince and I will soon reveal, the sit up is by no means the most effective abdominal exercise.

Right then, so what do we need to construct the perfect home gym?

Well, nothing really. If you have a set of dumbbells lying around the house that's great. In fact if you were to invest in one piece of equipment, make it a set of dumbells. They're dirt cheap, and can be used in literally dozens of exercises. But if you don't have any, it doesn't matter. The only advantage is added convenience, and we can easily improvise.

So here's what you will need:

1. Your own bodyweight.
2. A staircase.
3. 2 chairs.
4. Some plastic bottles or dumbbell weights.

5. A bed or sofa.
6. A broomstick handle.

The most important tool you have is yourself. Let's say, for example, if you have a bodyweight of 150 pounds, doing a press-up is similar to doing a 150-pound bench press at the gym. Doing pull-ups will be similar to using a pull-down machine stacked with 150 pounds of weight. It doesn't matter if you are unfamiliar with these exercises. The point is that we can use our bodyweight to help us.

The second most important thing we have is our intuition. We must be able to improvise in a way that will turn everyday objects around us into pieces of highly effective gym equipment. For example, if you take a 2-litre bottle and fill it to the top with water, it will weigh around two kilograms and become a two-kilogram dumbbell. A large book might weigh three to four kilograms. Pieces of furniture such as beds, chairs and sofas can be used as platforms to perform exercises on.

The 7-minute workout programme will show you how to utilise these everyday objects in order to sculpt the perfect body. If this seems a little far-fetched, bear with me. The following chapters will pull together all Vince Graham's secrets into a cohesive programme, which is going to transform the way you look.

CHAPTER FOUR
The Beginner's Workout

The Vince Graham 7 Minute A Day Body Sculpting Programme is highly effective in producing fast and effective results, but it's not as easy as the name might suggest. Although we only intend to exercise for 7 minutes per day, the activity that we are about to engage in is very intensive.

If you're new to exercise, or haven't done any for a while, I really wouldn't recommend that you dive straight in with the full-blown workout. You're probably going to find it too hard to go from doing nothing to doing this.

I think, if you're honest with yourself, you'll know whether you're ready to proceed to the full Vince Graham 7 Minute A Day Body Sculpting Programme. And if you are, feel free to skip this chapter and get stuck in. If you're in any doubt, I'd suggest you start with the three-day a week routine, and see how you feel on that first.

This three-day per week routine will develop some strength to prepare your body for Vince's system. This workout is structured in a way similar to those that you may find in health clubs... yes... I know, these programmes don't work very well, but this short one-month programme is not intended to carve the perfect body. It is merely here to get the body used to physical activity and develop a little strength.

This workout routine will last for seven minutes (similar to the Vince Graham workout) and is to be performed three times per week on Monday, Wednesday and Friday. Each session will involve training each of the major muscle groups for one minute. When I say the muscle groups are trained for one minute each, you must actually train for one minute. If after thirty seconds you need to rest, you can rest but you must perform the exercise for another thirty seconds after resting to ensure the exercise has been performed for a total of one minute. The correct order in which the exercises are to be performed is as follows:

1. Chest.
2. Back.
3. Shoulders.
4. Biceps.
5. Triceps.
6. Legs.
7. Abdominals.

It's important that you keep to this order. In fact, although this type of workout when performed in gyms and health clubs, doesn't work very well long term, it works a whole lot better when performed in this order.

I often see people working out in gyms in a totally haphazard manner, and usually with the blessing of their instructor! Triceps exercises are performed before chest exercises and biceps exercises are performed before those for the back. This is totally wrong and counter-productive.

The basic rule, when performing a routine which involves several muscle groups, is that you work the large muscle groups first before moving on to the smaller ones. Here's why…

Exercises for a large muscle group, like those of the chest, don't just involve that muscle group exclusively. So when you do a press up for example (which is primarily an exercise for the chest) the triceps at the rear of the arms are asked to do a lot of work. When you do a pull up (which is primarily an exercise for the back) your biceps have to work very hard.

Now…if you've worked your triceps before your chest, when you come to do your press ups it will be your triceps which give up first…because they're already tired. Why does this matter? Because your chest muscles don't get the work they need. They're just getting into their stride when your triceps give out.

It's exactly the same thing with your back and biceps. Work your biceps before doing some pull ups, and it will be your biceps that scream for mercy long before your back muscles have broken sweat.

So, always keep the golden rule in mind…large muscle groups come first!

The 3 Times A Week Workout

I just want to re-emphasise, this isn't The Vince Graham System, but it will help lay a foundation for you to build on later. If you're new to resistance exercise, even this routine might prove quite challenging at first, and it's certainly a lot better than most of the stuff being taught in health clubs.

Anyway, here's the routine…

Chest: The Press-up

This classic exercise strengthens the entire chest area and also works the shoulders and triceps as well.

1. Lie face down on the floor, supporting your weight on the balls of your feet and the palms of your hands. Your fingers should be pointing forwards and your hands should be slightly wider than shoulder width apart.
2. Maintain a straight line through your body by keeping your legs, back and neck straight. Keep your head facing the floor.
3. Slowly bend your arms, keeping the body straight, lowering the torso until it is about one inch away from the floor. Pause, and the return to the starting position.
4. Do not lock the elbows (to maintain continuous tension) and repeat the movement.

Please note: supporting your weight on your knees rather than the balls of the feet is an easier way of performing the exercise.

Back: Water Bottle One Arm Row

This move exercises the latissimus dorsi muscles as well as the rhomboids, adding both width and thickness to the back. The biceps are used as a secondary muscle. Use one two-litre or four-litre bottle filled with water as a weight.

1. Rest your left knee and left hand on a sofa, bed or chair. Plant your right foot firmly on the floor. Keep your back straight and your eyes facing the floor. Hold the bottle in your right hand, letting your right arm hand down with your palm facing towards you.
2. As though you are starting a lawnmower, pull the bottle up to your shoulder. Hold for a second, and then lower the bottle back again.
3. Perform this exercise for thirty seconds before switching sides and using the other arm for another thirty seconds.

Shoulders: Water Bottle Shoulder Press

This exercise requires the use of two bottles filled with water. This is the best exercise for the development of all portions of the deltoids. This exercise also works the triceps.

1. Sit in a chair with a reasonably upright backrest. Sit with your knees bent at ninety degrees and your feet planted on the floor. Hold one bottle in each hand at the sides of your shoulders.
2. Slowly press the bottles vertically above your head until your arms are almost straight. Then lower the bottles back to the starting position. Perform for one minute.

Biceps: Water Bottle Biceps Curls

If performed with strict adherence to correct form, this exercise will concentrate almost entirely on the biceps muscles. A pair of two-litre water bottles is required.

1. In a standing position (or seated in a chair), grasp two bottles by your sides, allowing your arms to hang down.
2. Keeping your elbows at your sides, with your upper arms stationary, curl the weights upwards towards the front of your shoulders. Then, in a controlled fashion, slowly lower them back down again. In order to ensure continuous tension, don't allow your arms to return to a fully extended position at the bottom. Perform the exercise for one minute.

Triceps: Water Bottle French Press Behind The Neck

This exercise works the triceps muscles and requires one two-litre bottle filled with water.

1. Grip the bottle at each end and lift it over your head. Keep your upper arms stationary either side of your head.
2. Slowly lower the bottle down behind your head until your arms are at an angle of ninety degrees. Then slowly press the weight back to the starting position. Perform the exercise for one minute.

Legs: Standing Squat

This is a great exercise for the quadriceps, hamstrings and buttocks.

1. Stand up straight with your legs at roughly shoulder-width apart. Keep your arms out of the way by placing your hands at the sides of your head.
2. Slowly bend the knees and lean the body forward slightly until the thighs are parallel to the floor. Pause for a moment and then raise your body back until your legs are almost straight.
3. Perform the exercise for one minute.

Abdominals: The Curl-up

The exercise is more effective than the sit-up as it maintains continuous tension and really works both the upper and lower abdominals.

1. Lie flat on your back with your knees bent at about 45 degrees and your arms crossed over your chest.
2. Curl your upper body forwards towards your knees, but unlike a sit up ensure that your lower back remains in contact with the floor. Try to raise the torso as high as possible by curling the body. At the top of the movement, really tense the abdominals for a second before returning to the starting position. To ensure continuous tension, don't let your shoulders touch the floor before performing another repetition. Focus your eyes at a point on the ceiling above your head for the duration of the exercise. Perform the exercise for one minute.

By now, you will have noticed that many of the exercises in Vince's system rely on you using your own bodyweight to help sculpt your body. Other exercises require the use of everyday objects to use as makeshift weights (usually bottles filled with water). If you feel it would be more convenient to use a proper set of dumbbells or you are finding the weights too light, you might consider buying a dumbbell set from your local sports shop. They are inexpensive and you may find them easier to work with.

If you decide to buy a set, I would recommend buying a set of dumbbells (usually you get three or four pairs) containing dumbbells weighing between 2.5kg and 10kg per dumbbell. A cheaper alternative is to buy a pair of dumbbell handles with either spring-clip or spin-lock collars and some weight plates. This way you can adjust the weight accordingly as you get stronger. If you are happy to improvise and use everyday objects for weights, that's also fine. You will be amazed at how easy it is to transform your home into the perfect gym.

After two or three weeks, you should notice some real improvement in strength and by the end of the fourth week you will be ready and prepared for the full intensity of the Vince Graham 7 Minute A Day Body Sculpting Programme. In the next chapter we will begin Vince's workout, so prepare yourself for some real improvements and get ready to start sculpting!

CHAPTER FIVE
The Full Workout – Monday: Chest

Now that we have sufficient knowledge about the body and how it works, I feel it's time to press on and transform that body. The time for theory is over, and the time for putting it into practice is about to begin in earnest.

In the following six chapters, you're going to learn in detail about the six muscle groups that we intend to transform, and exactly how we're going to do it.

Here's what you're going to be doing…and when:

1. Monday: Chest
2. Tuesday: Back
3. Wednesday: Shoulders
4. Thursday: Legs
5. Friday: Arms
6. Saturday: Abdominals
7. Sunday: Relax!

For each muscle group I will include the most effective exercises to target different parts of the muscle. I will also include stretching techniques to do prior to the workout to loosen the body and help avoid injury. I will then conclude each chapter with a proposed routine for each of the four weeks of the month. By having a different workout for each week of the month, we ensure constant change in order to maximise our improvement.

The Vince Graham System doesn't operate conventionally. If you've been exposed to regular gym and health club routines, you'll know what I mean by that – a routine made up of a number of sets and repetitions. The key to Vince's system is that you work for a fixed amount of time, rather than for a fixed number of sets and reps.

Sometimes, in order to make dramatic progress, you have to take dramatic action. Practically every resistance-training programme employs sets and repetitions as the core underlying principle. Vince worked out pretty early on, that the human body doesn't understand sets and repetitions. Nor does it respond to them.

The body only understands the amount of work it's being asked to perform, and the amount of time it's being given to perform that work. While sets and reps can be used to represent this work/time relationship, Vince's method effectively cuts out the middleman and addresses the relationship directly.

If you increase the work or shorten the time required to complete a given amount of work, then the exercise becomes more intense…or harder! When the body is subjected to demands it's not used to, (more intense exercise) it has to adapt, and those adaptations result in the body sculpting effect we're aiming for.

So, all the time, we're focusing on work and time…and the relationship between the two. Aside from the mirror and the tape measure, that's how we're going to be measuring progress.

If you're asked to perform an exercise for a period of time - a minute for example - and you are unable to continue after thirty seconds, you can rest for a while before performing the other thirty seconds. If you are given the target of performing one minute's worth of activity, you must complete one minute's worth of activity, even if it takes you six, ten second attempts.

Just to be clear though… your goal is to perform the exercise for the required amount of time in as few attempts as possible. Your ultimate goal is to be able to complete the full workout (7 minutes of exercise) in 7 minutes without resting. This will take a lot of time and effort but if Vince (at the age of 72!) can do it, so can you.

Monday: Chest Workout

Stretching

It's important to stretch the muscles prior to training them in order to warm them up for the gruelling exercises ahead. By stretching the muscles, you will help to prevent injuries such as pulled muscles, but you will also improve the quality of your workout because stretching is a good way of activating all of the muscle fibres.

A good way to warm up the pectoral muscles in the chest is to stand with your arms pointing straight out to your straight out to your sides (like the wings in a plane). Keeping your arms fairly straight swing your arms out in front of you, crossing them over and then back again until you can feel a comfortable stretching sensation in the chest area.

Another way to get a good stretch on the pectorals is to stand in a doorway (with the door open) and place one hand on each side of the doorframe. To stretch the muscles, simply push your body forwards, keeping your hands in contact with the doorframe.

The Chest Workout

The Press-up

This classic exercise strengthens the entire chest area and also works the shoulders and triceps as well.

1. Lie face down on the floor, supporting your weight on the balls of your feet and the palms of your hands. Your fingers should be pointing forwards and your hands should be slightly wider than shoulder width apart.

2. Maintain a straight line through your body by keeping your legs, back and neck straight. Keep your head facing the floor.

3. Slowly bend your arms, keeping the body straight, lowering the torso until it is about one inch away from the floor. Pause, and the return to the starting position.

4. Do not lock the elbows (to maintain continuous tension) and repeat the movement.

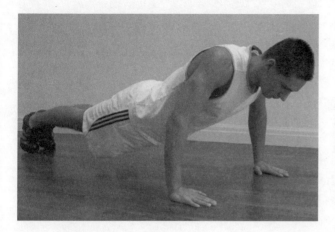 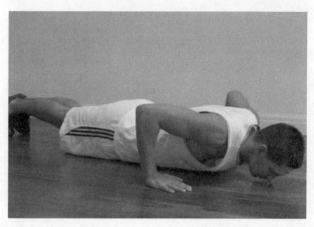

The Easy Press-up

This is an easier version of the press-up that may be a better when you first begin the programme just to develop your strength before attempting harder variations.

1. Lie face down on the floor, supporting your weight on your knees and the palms of your hands. Your fingers should be pointing forwards and your hands should be slightly wider than shoulder width apart.
2. Maintain a straight line through your body by keeping your legs, back and neck straight. Keep your head facing the floor.
3. Slowly bend your arms, keeping the body straight, lowering the torso until it is about one inch away from the floor. Pause, and the return to the starting position.
4. Do not lock the elbows (to maintain continuous tension) and repeat the movement.

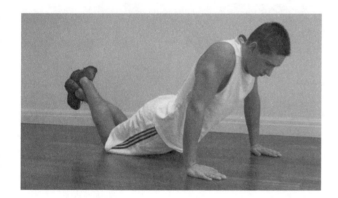 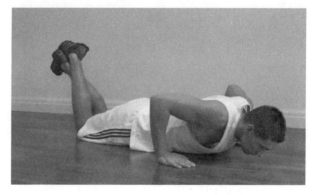

The Decline Press-up

This variation of the push-up is more difficult and focuses more on the upper portion of the pectorals.

1. With your feet raised above head level either on a chair or on the first or second step of your staircase, lie face down, supporting your weight on the balls or instep of your feet and the palms of your hands. Your fingers should be pointing forwards and your hands should be slightly wider than shoulder width apart.
2. Maintain a straight line through your body by keeping your legs, back and neck straight. Keep your head facing the floor.

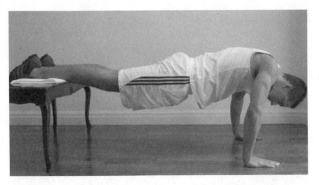 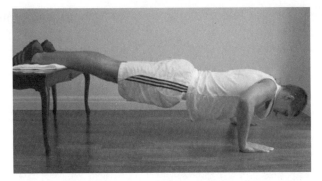

3. Slowly bend your arms, keeping the body straight, lowering the torso until it is about one inch away from the floor. Pause, and the return to the starting position.
4. Do not lock the elbows (to maintain continuous tension) and repeat the movement.

The Incline Press-up

This variation of the push-up is slightly easier and focuses more on the lower portion of the pectorals.

1. With your hands raised above head level either on a chair or on the first or second step of your staircase, lie facedown, supporting your weight on the balls of your feet and the palms of your hands. Your fingers should be pointing forwards or grasping the sides of the chair and your hands should be about shoulder width apart.
2. Maintain a straight line through your body by keeping your legs, back and neck straight. Keep your head facing the floor.
3. Slowly bend your arms, keeping the body straight, lowering the torso until it is about one inch away from the floor. Pause, and the return to the starting position.
4. Do not lock the elbows (to maintain continuous tension) and repeat the movement.

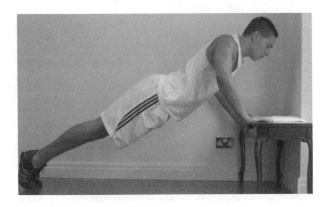 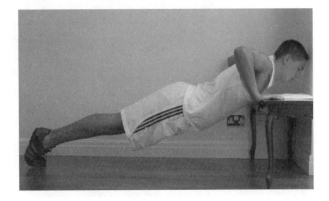

The Jump Press-up or Clap Press-up

This press-up emphasises the use of explosive power in the positive portion of the exercise. The exercise is much more difficult and should be performed only when your strength is further developed.

1. Lie face down on the floor, supporting your weight on the balls of your feet and the palms of your hands. Your fingers should be pointing forwards and your hands should be slightly wider than shoulder width apart.
2. Maintain a straight line through your body by keeping your legs, back and neck straight. Keep your head facing the floor.

3. Slowly bend your arms, keeping the body straight, lowering the torso until it is about one inch away from the floor.
4. Pause at the bottom and then using explosive power, push your body up, bringing your hands away from the floor (you may clap them if you wish) before catching yourself by returning your palms to the floor.

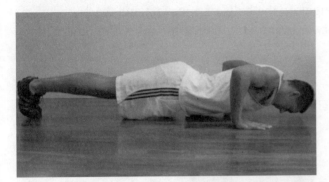 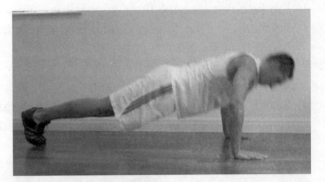

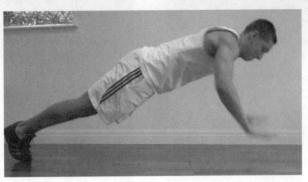

The Wide Grip Press-up

This exercise is similar to the classic press-up but emphasises the outer portion of the pectoral muscles. The easy version of the press-up can also be performed with a wider grip.

1. Lie face down on the floor, supporting your weight on the balls of your feet and the palms of your hands. Your fingers should be pointing forwards and your hands should be much wider than shoulder width apart.
2. Maintain a straight line through your body by keeping your legs, back and neck straight. Keep your head facing the floor.
3. Slowly bend your arms, keeping the body straight, lowering the torso until it is about one inch away from the floor. Pause, and the return to the starting position.
4. Do not lock the elbows (to maintain continuous tension) and repeat the movement.

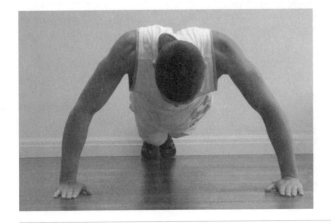 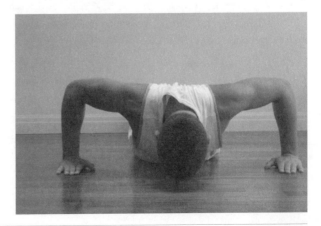

The Close Grip Press-up

This movement is similar to the classic press-up but emphasises the inner portion of the pectoral muscles. This exercise also puts slightly more emphasis on the triceps.

1. Lie face down on the floor, supporting your weight on the balls of your feet and the palms of your hands. Your fingers should be pointing forwards and your hands should be slightly narrower than shoulder width apart.
2. Maintain a straight line through your body by keeping your legs, back and neck straight. Keep your head facing the floor.
3. Slowly bend your arms, keeping the body straight, lowering the torso until it is about one inch away from the floor. Pause, and the return to the starting position.
4. Do not lock the elbows (to maintain continuous tension) and repeat the movement.

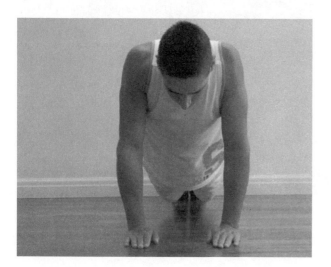 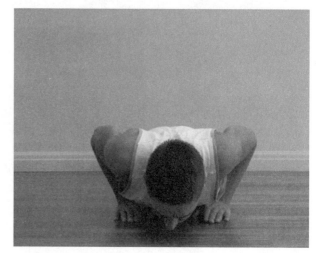

The Water Bottle Fly

This exercise works all portions of the pectoral muscles and also works the front of the shoulders. As your strength develops, you can add more water to the bottles or use larger bottles or even books.

1. Lie on your back on a bench or footstool with your legs parted for balance and your feet firmly on the floor. Hold two water bottles above your with your palms facing each other.

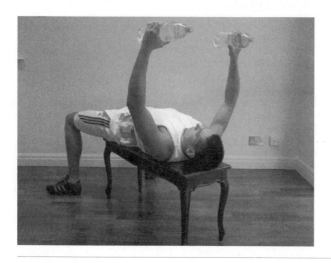 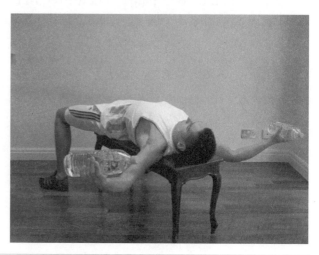

2. Lower the bottles down to shoulder level with your arms slightly bent at the elbows. The arms should move in an arc-like movement.
3. Raise your arms back above you.
4. It is better not to touch the bottles together at the top, but to leave a gap of around 10 inches between them in order to maintain continuous tension on the muscles.

Suggested Chest Routines

To ensure continuous improvement, it is important to keep changing the routine so that the body does not grow accustomed to carrying out the same routine. We will ensure constant change by using different combinations of exercises and also by utilising the various core techniques of the Vince Graham System (supersets, super slow, explosive power and so on).

Please note that prior to starting the workout, it is advisable to spend a few minutes stretching or even warming up by jogging on the spot or going for a brisk walk.

Week One: The Superset Program

A great method that Vince incorporates into his system is a technique used by bodybuilders known as the 'Superset'. For more information on this, you can refer back to the section on supersets in Chapter 2.

Vince stresses that the key to the 7-minute workout is intensity. Supersets allow us to maximise the amount of work that we can achieve in 7 minutes.

As we know, super-setting involves combining two or more exercises for the same muscle group. The goal here is pre-exhaustion. A pre-exhaust superset is performed by choosing two exercises for the same muscle group. An isolation exercise first, followed by a basic, compound movement. Remember, compound exercises are exercises that are intended to train a particular muscle but also train other muscles as secondary muscles. Isolation exercises on the other hand are exercises that focus entirely on one muscle and do not involve any other muscles as secondary muscles.

The principle of 'pre-exhaustion' utilises isolation and compound movements in such a way as to make the compound movements more effective in working the target muscle group.

In this instance, we will be using the pre-exhaustion principle to increase the effectiveness of the Press-up movements. To achieve this, we must partially tire (pre-exhaust) the pectorals before performing the compound movements. Performing an isolation exercise such as Water Bottle Flys before the compound movements, can achieve this.

Other workouts in the Vince Graham system require you to perform a particular exercise for a fixed amount of time (for example, one minute). The superset programme will differ from the other workouts in that you will be required to perform a particular exercise to exhaustion before performing a different exercise.

Here's why...

The underlying goal of performing a superset is to eliminate all rest periods for the duration of the set. If you were asked to perform Decline Press-ups for 2 minutes non-stop, I am pretty sure that you would find that exhausting… certainly far too exhausting to be in a position to complete a further set of another exercise immediately afterwards without rest. So here's what we'll do...

In the superset routine, your goal will be to perform each exercise to failure (until your final repetition results in failure – you just can't lift it). Then, as soon as you fail to perform the final repetition on the first exercise, you must progress immediately to the second exercise and perform that exercise to failure too. And so on until you have completed the four exercises in the superset.

Upon completion of the superset, you will be allowed a short amount of time to rest (30-60 seconds) before commencing the superset for a second time. Your goal is to continue with the process until you have completed 7 minutes of activity. And here's the bad news – you are not allowed to count the rest period (30-60 seconds) between supersets as part of the total 7 minutes!

Here are the exercises for the chest routine – and the order to do them in.

1. Water Bottle Flys, performed to failure.
2. Incline Press-ups, performed to failure.
3. Water Bottle Flys, performed to failure.
4. Decline Press-ups, performed to failure.

*IMPORTANT NOTE: Remember, you should not rest between performing these exercises. You should aim to only rest upon completion of a 'round' of these exercises for a period of 30 to 60 seconds before repeating the superset.

Week Two: The Explosive Power Program

The explosive power programme will really help to develop strength by over emphasising the positive portion of the exercise. The positive portion should be performed with speed and power and the negative portion performed at normal speed.

1. Perform Wide Grip Jump Press-ups for 2 minutes.
2. Perform Incline Jump Press-ups for 2 minutes.
3. Perform Water Bottle Flys for 3 minutes.*

*When performing the water bottle flys, raise the bottles above you with more speed than usual and lower them down with less speed.

Week Three: The Negatives Programme

When performing exercises using the negatives method, it is important to perform the negative portion of the exercise slowly but the positive portion at the normal speed.

1. Perform the classic press-up emphasising the negative portion for 2 minutes.
2. Perform the close-grip press-up emphasising the negative portion for 2 minutes.
3. Perform the decline press-up emphasising the negative portion for 1 minute.
4. Perform water bottle flys for 2 minutes emphasising the negative portion.

Week 4: The Super-Slow Programme

The super-slow method is very difficult and involves performing each repetition for roughly ten seconds. Five seconds for the positive and five seconds for the negative portion of the exercise. Because of the increased level of difficulty, you may wish to perform the push-up exercises in the 'easy' style by supporting your weight on the knees rather than the balls of the feet.

1. Perform the classic press-up for 1 minute.
2. Perform water bottle flys for 2 minutes.
3. Perform incline press-ups for 1 minute.
4. Perform wide grip press-ups for 1 minute.
5. Perform close-grip press-ups for 1 minute.
6. Perform water bottle flys a second time for 1 minute.

CHAPTER SIX
Tuesday: Back Workout

Stretching

As with the chest muscles, to avoid injury, you need to ensure that you gently stretch the back muscles before you train them.

One good way to stretch the muscles in the upper back is to simply grab hold of a piece of furniture or door frame with one hand and pull until you feel a stretching sensation in your back muscles. Make sure that you feel this sensation in both sides of the back by changing the hand you use to hold the object.

An alternative to this stretching movement is to hold onto something overhead and hang with your feet off the floor, supporting your weight with your hands. By doing this, your back muscles are stretched by the weight of your body.

The above two exercises are to focus the stretch in the upper back. To properly stretch the lower back muscles, you need to lie flat on the floor, facedown. Slowly push your upper body off the floor until your arms are straight. Your hips and legs should remain in contact with the floor so that the movement arches the back.

The Back Workout

Water Bottle One Arm Row

This move exercises the latissimus dorsi muscles as well as the rhomboids, adding both width and thickness to the back. The biceps are used as a secondary muscle. Use one two-litre or four-litre bottle filled with water as a weight.

1. Rest your left knee and left hand on a sofa, bed or chair. Plant your right foot firmly on the floor. Keep your back straight and your eyes facing the floor. Hold the bottle in your right hand, letting your right arm hand down with your palm facing towards you.

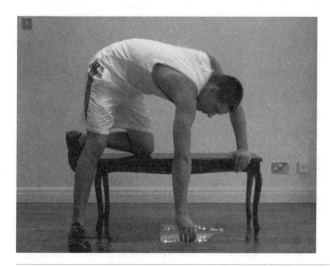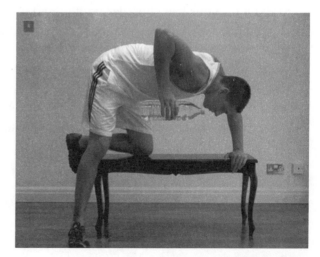

2. As though you are starting a lawnmower, pull the bottle up to your shoulder. Hold for a second, and then lower the bottle back again. To ensure continuous tension, do not fully extend the arm at the bottom of the movement.
3. Perform this exercise for thirty seconds before switching sides and using the other arm for another thirty seconds.

Water Bottle Rowing

This move exercises the same muscles as the 'one-arm row', but enables you to work both sides of the back at the same time.

1. Lie facedown on a bench. Grasp two water-filled bottles and allow them to hang down until they almost touch the floor. Your palms should be facing inwards.
2. Slowly raise the bottles in a count of two up to shoulder level, hold for a second before lowering them back to starting position. Again, ensure continuous tension by eliminating the rest period at the bottom portion of the exercise.

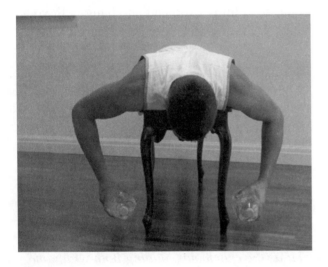 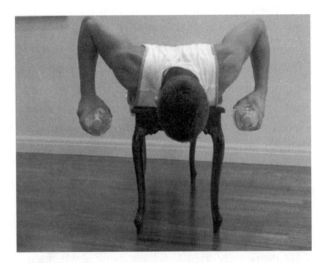

Standing Water Bottle Rowing

This exercise works the back and biceps muscles as well as the hamstrings, rear deltoids, gluteal muscles and abs.

1. Stand with your feet shoulder width apart and your knees slightly bent.
2. Bend at the waist until your upper body is straight and parallel to the floor. Hold two water filled bottles (two or four litres each) at arms length with your hands farther than shoulder width apart and your palms facing your body.
3. Raise the bottles in a count of two until your elbows are higher than your back. Your forearms should be perpendicular to the floor. Hold for a second, then slowly lower the bottles to about mid-shin level, and repeat. Avoid fully extending the arms to ensure that we achieve a peak contraction through continuous tension.

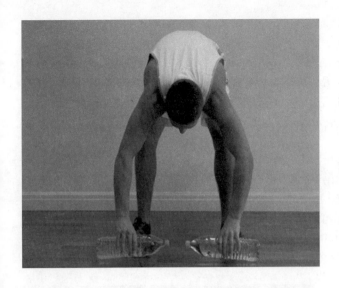
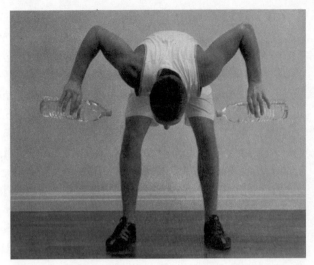

Chins

This exercise is the single best exercise for developing the upper back muscles and is a great way to achieve the 'V' shaped look. Most homes will have somewhere where you can perform this exercise. You can purchase a 'chinning bar' which fits easily into a domestic doorway for just a few pounds, or failing that I would suggest using a staircase, child's swing or climbing frame to perform this exercise. Safety Note: It is essential that you ensure whatever you're using is strong and stable enough to support your weight during the movement.

This is a very difficult movement and should only be attempted when you have developed your strength in the biceps and back muscles.

1. Grasp an object overhead with your hands slightly wider than shoulder width apart.
2. You should hang with your arms fully extended to achieve a good stretch in the back muscles.
3. From this position, slowly pull your body up until your chin is level with your hands. Pause for a moment and then lower yourself back to the starting position.

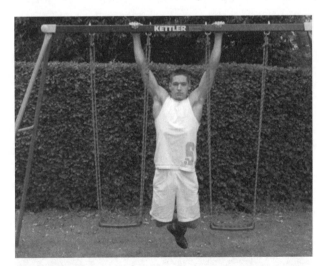
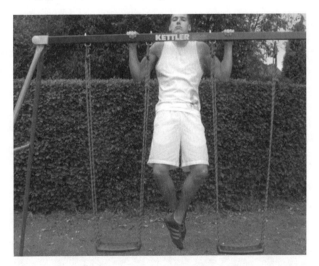

4. With chinning exercises, Vince believes that getting a good stretch at the bottom of the exercise is beneficial and therefore you don't need to worry too much about continuous tension. I would suggest stretching at the bottom for less than a second in duration however, just to avoid over-resting the muscles.

Wide Grip Chins

This exercise is a variation on the classic chin illustrated above. By utilising a wider grip, the exercise becomes harder but more focused on the back muscles. Most homes will have somewhere where you can perform this exercise. This is a very difficult movement and should only be attempted when you have developed your strength in the biceps and back muscles.

1. Grasp an object overhead with your hands slightly wider than shoulder width apart. I would suggest using a staircase or child's swing or climbing frame to perform this exercise.
2. You should hang with your arms fully extended to achieve a good stretch in the back muscles.
3. From this position, slowly pull your body up until your chin is level with your hands. Pause for a moment and then lower yourself back to the starting position. In the same manner as with classic chins, a good stretch at the bottom of the exercise is beneficial to its effectiveness.

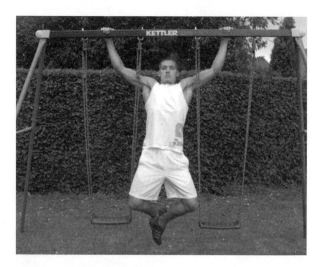 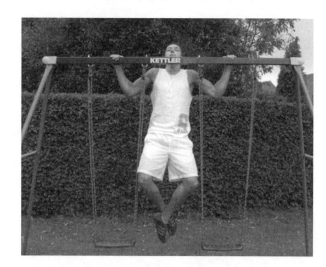

Water Bottle Pullovers

This exercise is an isolation exercise for the latissimus dorsi muscles in the upper back. To perform this exercise, you will require one heavy, water-filled bottle.

1. Lie across a bench with only your shoulders and upper back in contact with the bench. Your legs should be shoulder width apart, feet planted firmly and your shins should be perpendicular to the floor.

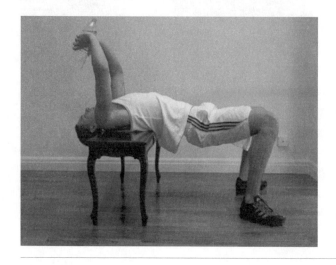 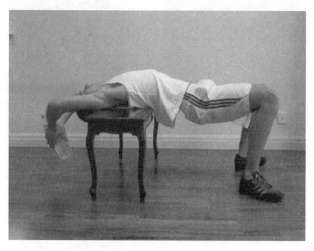

2. Grasp the bottle in both hands above your head.
3. Slowly lower the bottle behind your head, keeping your arms slightly bent until it almost touches the floor. Pause for a moment and return the weight back again. At the top of the movement, you should reduce the range of motion to ensure constant tension on the lats.

Suggested Back Routines

To ensure continuous improvement, it is important to keep changing the routine so that the body does not grow accustomed to carrying out the same routine. As with the chest routine, we will ensure constant change by using different combinations of exercises and also by utilising the various core techniques of the Vince Graham System (supersets, super slow, explosive power and so on).

Please note that prior to starting the workout, it is advisable to spend a few minutes stretching or even warming up by jogging on the spot or going for a brisk walk.

Week One: The Superset Program

A great method that Vince incorporates into his system is a technique used by bodybuilders known as the 'Superset'. For more information on this, you can refer back to the section on supersets in Chapter 2.

As you already are aware, to increase the effectiveness of a compound movement, we must use an isolation exercise to pre-exhaust the target muscle group. In this instance, we will be using the Water Bottle Pullovers as a pre-exhaustion exercise for the latissimus dorsi muscles before performing the compound movements for the upper back.

The compound movements we will be using are Chins and Standing Water Bottle Rows. I chose this combination of compound movements because Chins are the single most effective exercise for adding width to the back. Chinning movements are essential to that 'V' shaped torso. I also included a rowing movement as I feel the Standing Water Bottle Row complements the chinning movement well because it focuses on thickness rather than width.

You will be required to perform each exercise to failure (until your final repetition results in failure – you just can't lift it). Then, as soon as you fail to perform the final repetition on the first exercise, you must progress immediately to the second exercise and perform the exercise to failure. And so on until you have completed the four exercises in the superset.

Upon completion of the superset, you will be allowed a short amount of time to rest (30-60 seconds) before commencing the superset for a second time. You must continue with the process until you have completed 7 minutes of activity. And here's the bad news – you are not allowed to count the rest period (30-60 seconds) between supersets as part of the total 7 minutes.

Listed below is the order in which you must complete the exercises for the back superset:

1. Water Bottle Pullovers, performed to failure.
2. Chins, performed to failure.
3. Water Bottle Pullovers, performed to failure.
4. Standing Water Bottle Rowing, performed to failure.

*IMPORTANT NOTE: Remember, you must not rest between performing the different exercises listed above. You can only rest upon completion of these exercises for a period of 30 to 60 seconds before repeating the superset.

Week Two: The Explosive Power Program

The explosive power programme will really help to develop strength by over emphasising the positive portion of the exercise. The positive portion should be performed with speed and power and the negative portion performed at normal speed.

1. Perform Wide Grip Chins for 1 minute, putting speed into pulling the body up.
2. Perform Water Bottle Rowing for 3 minutes.
3. Perform water bottle one arm rows for 2 minutes.
4. Perform standing water bottle rowing for 1 minute. .

*Perform lying back extensions at normal speed and power. Explosive movements for this exercise are likely to result in injury.

Week Three: The Negatives Programme

When performing exercises using the negatives method, it is important to perform the negative portion of the exercise slowly but the positive portion at the normal speed.

1. Perform the classic chins emphasising the negative portion for 1 minute.
2. Perform standing water bottle rowing emphasising the negative portion for 2 minutes.
3. Perform water bottle one-arm rows for 2 minutes emphasising the negative portion (one-minute per arm).
4. Perform water bottle pullovers for 2 minutes.

Week 4: The Super-Slow Programme

The super-slow method is very difficult and involves performing each repetition for roughly ten seconds. Five seconds for the positive and five seconds for the negative portion of the exercise. Because of the increased level of difficulty, I have excluded the 'chinning' exercises from this routine. If you feel that you are strong enough to perform chins in super slow, by all means you may adapt the programme to include them. Alternatively, you may include them but perform them at normal speed.

1. Perform the water bottle rowing for 2 minutes.
2. Perform lying back extensions for 2 minutes.
3. Perform standing water bottle rowing for 1 minute.
4. Perform one-arm water bottle rowing for 2 minutes (one minute for each arm).

CHAPTER SEVEN
Wednesday: Shoulder Workout

Stretching

The shoulders are one of the most commonly injured body parts, so it is very important to ensure that they are properly warmed up before performing these exercises. This stretching routine is highly effective in preparing the shoulders for intense exercise:

1. Rotate both arms forwards for 30 seconds as though swimming and performing the front crawl but rotate both arms at the same time instead of one then the other.
2. Rotate them backwards for 30 seconds.
3. Clasp your fingers together with your palms facing away from you and stretch your arms out in front of you. Hold for 10 seconds.
4. With your arms in this position, raise them above your head and hold for 10 seconds.
5. Clasp your hands together behind your back with palms facing each other. Gently raise your arms behind you until you feel a comfortable stretch.
6. Loosen off the shoulders by rolling your shoulders forwards for 30 seconds with your arms by your sides.
7. Roll your shoulders backwards for 30 seconds.

Your shoulders should now be sufficiently warmed up to perform the following exercises.

The Shoulder Workout

Water Bottle Shoulder Press

This exercise is the best for developing the entire area of the deltoid muscle group. The triceps are also worked in the movement. This exercise can be performed either seated or standing. If performed in a seated position, you must sit up straight with your back perpendicular to the floor.

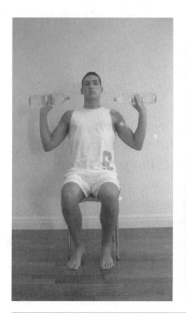 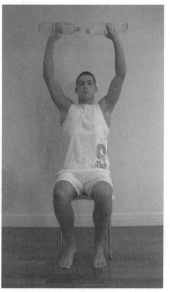

1. In either a seated or standing position, grasp two bottles at head height at either side of your shoulders. Your hands should be positioned with your palms facing away from your head.
2. To perform the exercise, slowly press the water bottles up and above your head until your arms are almost straight. Pause for a moment before returning to the starting position. Repeat.

Water Bottle Arnold Press

This exercise is a variation of the classic shoulder press utilises the rotation of the wrists to focus the benefit on different areas of the deltoids. As you may have guessed, it was developed by seven-time Mr. Olympia, movie star, and politician... Gvnr. Arnold Schwarzenegger.

1. This exercise may be performed in either a seated or standing position, adopting a similar stance to the classic shoulder press movement.
2. Grasp the bottles in front of the chest this time with your palms facing towards you.
3. Slowly press the bottles above your head whilst rotating the wrist towards each other so that

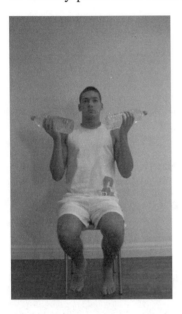 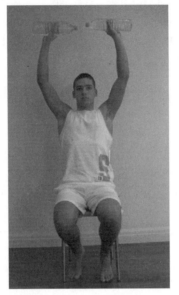

halfway through the movement, your palms are facing each other.

4. Continue to press the bottles until your arms are almost straight whilst rotating the wrists further until your palms are facing away from you. Pause before lowering the bottles to the starting position.

5. As you lower the bottles, rotate the wrists back again so that when you return to the starting position, your palms are once again facing towards your chest. When you return to the starting position, do not pause. Press the weight immediately to ensure continuous tension.

Water Bottle Side Lateral Raise

This exercise works the side deltoids, adding width to your shoulders. By developing these muscles, your upper body will appear broader and your waist will appear slimmer.

1. Because this movement focuses only on the side deltoids (a small muscle), you may need to use

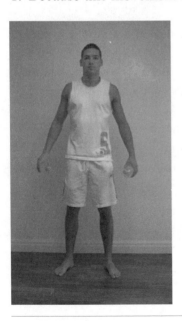 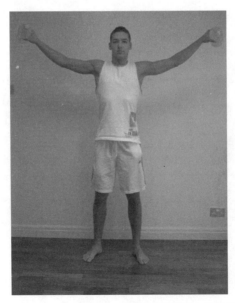

smaller bottles or you can simply pour some water out of your two litre bottles.

2. Stand up straight with your feet about shoulder width apart with your knees unlocked. You should hold the bottles at your sides with your elbows slightly bent and your palms facing towards your sides.

3. To perform the exercise, raise the bottles up to head height. You should keep the elbows slightly bent and avoid rotating the wrists. At the top of the

movement, your palms should be facing the floor.

4. Pause for a moment before lowering the bottles. Repeat.
5. When you lower the bottles, lower them to a point about ten inches from your sides to ensure that the resting period at the lower portion of the exercise is eliminated. You should also adopt this approach when performing the following lateral and front raise exercises...

Advanced Water Bottle Side Lateral Raise

This is a variation of the classic side lateral raise that utilises wrist rotation to include the other areas of the deltoid muscles.

1. Again, you may need to use smaller bottles or lighter bottles.
2. Stand up straight with your feet about shoulder width apart with your knees unlocked. You should hold the bottles at your sides with your elbows slightly bent but this time with your palms facing forwards and your thumb pointing towards the roof.
3. To perform the exercise, raise the bottles up to head height. You should keep the elbows slightly bent and rotate the wrists forwards for the duration of the exercise. Half way through the movement, your palms should face the floor with your thumb pointing forwards. At the top of the movement, your palms should be facing behind you with your thumb pointing to the floor.
4. When performing the movement, imagine the lids are off the bottles and you are pouring the water out as you raise your arms to head level.
5. Pause for a moment before lowering the bottles. As you lower the bottles, you should rotate the wrists back again. Repeat.

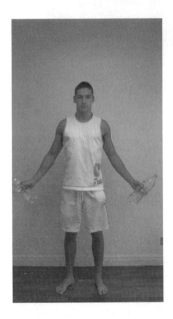 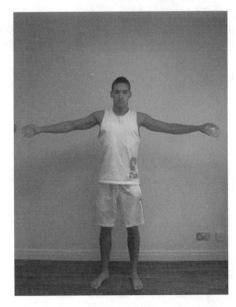 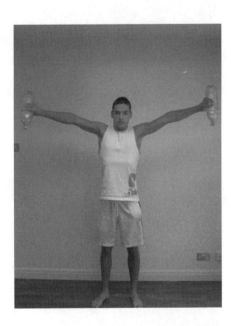

Standing, Alternating Front Raises

This exercise focuses more on the front deltoids and also involves the upper chest slightly. As with the lateral raises, you may require lighter weights.

1. Adopt a standing position with your feet approximately shoulder width apart. Hold the bottles at your sides with your elbows slightly bent as thought about to perform a lateral raise.
2. Slowly raise the bottle in your left hand up in front of you to head level. The palm of your hand should be facing the floor. Pause for a moment and then lower to the starting position.
3. Repeat the movement with the other arm, return to starting position. Repeat.

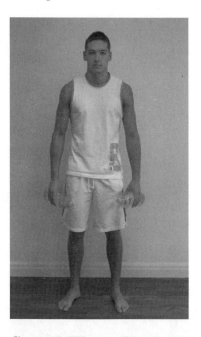 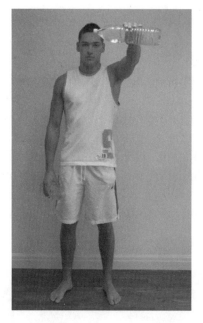 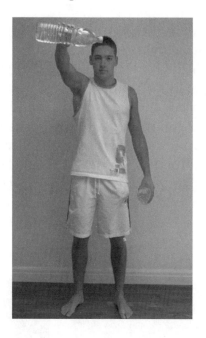

Seated Water Bottle Front Raises

This exercise focuses more on the front deltoids and also involves the upper chest slightly. As with the lateral raises, you may require lighter weights.

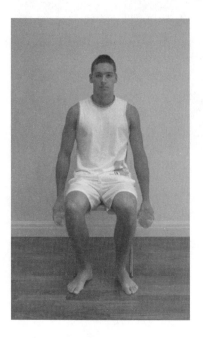 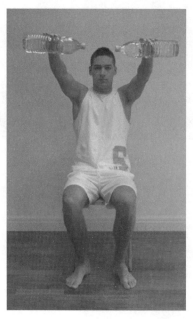

1. Adopt a seated position with your feet planted firmly on the floor approximately shoulder width apart. You should sit as upright as possible with your back perpendicular to the floor. Hold the bottles at your sides with your elbows slightly bent as thought about to perform a lateral raise.
2. Slowly raise both bottles up in front of you to head level. At the top of the movement, the palms of your hands should be facing the floor. Pause for a moment and then lower to the starting position. Repeat.

Rear Deltoid Water Bottle Raise

This movement focuses on the rear deltoid muscles and should be performed with light bottles of water. You will need a chair and a towel to perform this exercise.

1. Adopt a standing position behind the chair with your feet approximately shoulder width apart.

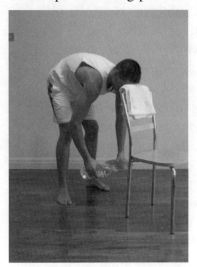 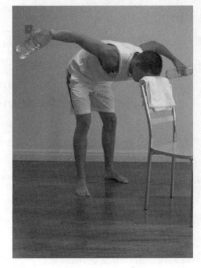

Bend over to rest your forehead on the backrest of the chair. Use the towel for padding to make the exercise more comfortable.

2.   Hold the water bottles below you, allowing your arms to hang down.

3.   Slowly raise the bottles in a semi-circular motion up to shoulder level with your elbows slightly bent. Your palms should be facing the floor. At the top of the movement, pause for a moment before lowering the bottles back to the starting position. Repeat.

Seated Rear Deltoid Raise

This movement is an alternative to the exercise described above. It also focuses on the rear deltoids. You should experiment to find out which exercise is most comfortable or perform both to add variety to the programme.

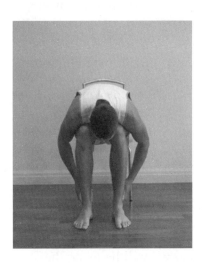 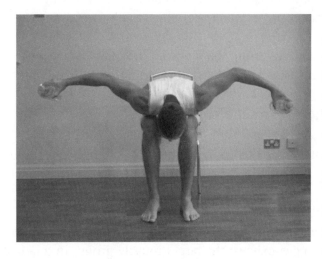

1.Adopt a seated position at the end of a bench. You should be hunched over with your chest almost touching your knees. Your feet should be together and firmly planted on the floor.

2. Start the movement with the bottles below your legs. Slowly raise the bottles to shoulder level, pause for a moment and return to the starting position. Repeat.

Upright Water Bottle Row

This exercise focuses on the trapezius muscles and also uses the biceps as a secondary muscle.

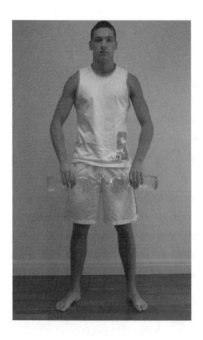 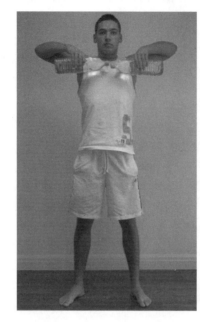

1.   Adopt a standing position with feet shoulder width apart and knees unlocked. Hold a bottle in each hand in front of your thighs with your palms facing your legs.
2.   Slowly raise the bottles to chin height, keeping your palms facing towards your body. Pause for a moment, before returning to the starting position. Repeat.
3.   This exercise could also be performed with one large bottle grasped in both hands or also you could use a briefcase or light chair.
4.   Please take care not to fully extend the arms at the lower portion of the exercise to ensure continuous tension.

Suggested Shoulder Routines

To ensure continuous improvement, it is important to keep changing the routine so that the body does not grow accustomed to carrying out the same routine. We will ensure constant change by using different combinations of exercises and also by utilising the various core techniques of the Vince Graham System (supersets, super slow, explosive power and so on).

Please note that prior to starting the workout, it is advisable to spend a few minutes stretching or even warming up by jogging on the spot or going for a brisk walk.

Week One: The Superset Program

A great method that Vince incorporates into his system is a technique used by bodybuilders known as the 'Superset'. For more information on this, you can refer back to the section on supersets in Chapter 2.

As you already are aware, to increase the effectiveness of a compound movement, we must use an isolation exercise to pre-exhaust the target muscle group. In this instance, we will be using the Water Bottle Front Raises and Seated Rear Deltoid Raises as pre-exhaustion exercises for the front and rear deltoid muscles respectively.

These isolation exercises will be combined with the Classic Shoulder Press and the Arnold Press, which are compound movements since they also work the triceps and upper chest. The compound movements will become much more effective as shoulder exercises following the pre-exhaustion of the front and rear deltoids.

You will be required to perform each exercise to failure (until your final repetition results in failure – you just can't lift it). Then, as soon as you fail to perform the final repetition on the first exercise, you must progress immediately to the second exercise and perform the exercise to failure. And so on until you have completed the four exercises in the superset.

Upon completion of the superset, you will be allowed a short amount of time to rest (30-60 seconds) before commencing the superset for a second time. You must continue with the process until you have completed 7 minutes of activity. And here's the bad news – you are not allowed to count the rest period (30-60 seconds) between supersets as part of the total 7 minutes.

Listed below is the order in which you must completed the exercises for the shoulder superset:

1. Water Bottle Front Raises, performed to failure.
2. Classic Water Bottle Shoulder Press, performed to failure.
3. Seated Rear Deltoid Raises, performed to failure.
4. Water Bottle Arnold Press, performed to failure.

*IMPORTANT NOTE: Remember, you must not rest between performing the different exercises listed above. You can only rest upon completion of these exercises for a period of 30 to 60 seconds before repeating the superset.

Week Two: The Explosive Power Program

The explosive power programme will really help to develop strength by over emphasising the positive portion of the exercise. The positive portion should be performed with speed and power and the negative portion performed at normal speed.

1. Perform the Water Bottle Shoulder Press for 2 minutes.
2. Perform Standing, Alternating Front Raises for 2 minutes.
3. Perform the Standing Rear Deltoid Raise for 2 minutes.
4. Perform the Upright Water Bottle Row for 1 minute.

Week Three: The Negatives Programme

When performing exercises using the negatives method, it is important to perform the negative portion of the exercise slowly but the positive portion at the normal speed.

1. Perform the Water Bottle Arnold Press emphasising the negative portion for 2 minutes.
2. Perform the classic Lateral Water Bottle Raise emphasising the negative portion for 2 minutes.
3. Perform the Water Bottle Upright Row emphasising the negative portion for 1 minute.
4. Perform the Standing Rear Deltoid Raise for 2 minutes emphasising the negative portion.

Week 4: The Super-Slow Programme

The super-slow method is very difficult and involves performing each repetition for roughly ten seconds. Five seconds for the positive and five seconds for the negative portion of the exercise. Super slow movements are highly effective because the duration of the exercise ensures that all the muscle fibres are fully engaged, resulting in 'peak contraction'.

1. Perform the Classic Shoulder Press for 1 minute.
2. Perform Water Bottle Side Lateral Raises for 1 minute.
3. Perform Water Bottle Arnold Presses for 1 minute.
4. Perform Advanced Water Bottle Lateral Raises for 1 minute.
5. Perform Standing, Alternating Front Raises for 1 minute.
6. Perform Rear Deltoid Water Bottle Raises for 1 minute.
7. Perform Upright Water Bottle Rows for 1 minute.

CHAPTER EIGHT
Thursday: Legs and Buttocks Workout

I've spent a lot of time in gyms and seen a lot of neglected legs. For many men, their primary concern is a large chest and big arms. Legs are unimportant... something for hiding in jeans and standing on. This is a big mistake, which usually comes 'home to roost' on the beach or at the pool.

Women on the other hand, are self-conscious about every body part. Their legs are often on display, and they want them to look good. But they simply don't know the correct way to train them. They spend hours on treadmills and cycling machines, but achieve very little in terms of aesthetic improvement. They are wary about using resistance exercises because they think they're going to build 'full back's' thighs.

The upshot is that very few people...male or female...train their legs properly.

In this section we'll be focusing on a combination of lower body exercises and techniques, which will enable you to create perfectly toned, defined legs and a 'toned tush' as well.

Stretching

The following stretching exercises will prepare your legs for the intense workout to come. Follow the instructions carefully as correct stretching will help to avoid injury and also improve the quality of the workout.

1. Groin stretch: Sit on the floor with your legs bent and the soles of your feet pressed together. Press your knees down as close to the floor as possible using the muscles in your legs only. Hold for 10 seconds. Then, grasp your ankles and press down on the knees with your elbows. Hold for 15 seconds.
2. Hamstring stretch: Stand up straight with your feet together. Slowly bend at the waist, keeping your legs straight, reach down and try to touch your toes. Do not bounce with your bodyweight as this often results in injuries. Hold at the bottom for 15 seconds and return to the starting position. Repeat once more.
3. Thigh stretch: Stand, holding a piece of furniture or wall for support. Bend your right knee and grab your right foot with your right hand, pulling your foot so it presses against your buttocks. Hold for a moment, and then switch legs. Repeat once more.
4. Calf stretch: Stand upright. Move your right leg in front of your left leg, keeping both feet pointing forwards. Bend the right leg, and keep the left leg straight with the heel of your left foot on the floor. Continue until you feel a comfortable stretch in the calf of your left leg. Hold, switch legs and repeat.

The Leg Workout

Standing Squat

This exercise strengthens your thighs as well as your gluteal muscles and lower back. This exercise is convenient and can be performed anywhere. To add resistance to the movement, you can support water bottles on your shoulders.

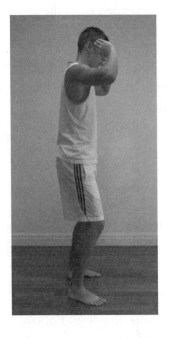
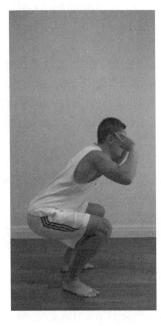

1. Adopt a standing position with your feet approximately shoulder width apart. Place your hands at the sides of your temples if using no weight. If you intend to use water bottles to add resistance, you can use your hands to support the bottles on your shoulders.

2. From this position, bend at the knees and lower your body down until your thighs are parallel to the floor. You may lean your torso forward slightly as you lower down, but ensure that the spine remains straight to avoid injury.

3. At the bottom of the movement, pause for a moment before pressing the body back up again. To ensure continuous tension, do not return to a fully standing position. Ensure the legs remain slightly bent, even at the top of the movement. Repeat.

The Single Leg Squat

This is a much harder (well twice as hard actually) version of the standing squat. You will struggle to perform the exercise for as long. You will need the support of a piece of furniture for balance.

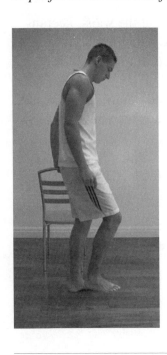
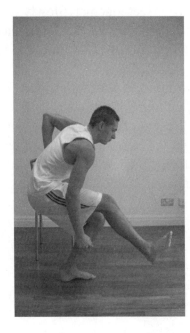

1. Stand upright with your feet shoulder width apart and your knees slightly bent. Place your left hand on a piece of furniture and your right hand on your hip for balance.

2. Slowly begin to squat on your left leg while extending your right leg out in front of you. You must keep your back straight through the entire movement. As soon as your left thigh is parallel to the floor, press your body back up again.

3. In order to maintain continuous tension, ensure that the knee remains partially bent at the top of the movement. Perform until fatigued, then switch legs.

The Squat Jump

This exercise strengthens your thighs as well as your gluteal muscles and lower back. This exercise is a variation of the standing squat but utilises an explosive movement.

1. Adopt a standing position with your feet approximately shoulder width apart. Place your hands on your temples..
2. From this position, bend at the knees and lower your body down until your thighs are parallel to the floor. You may lean your torso forward slightly as you lower down, but ensure that the spine remains straight to avoid injury.
3. At the bottom of the movement, use explosive power to jump your feet away from the ground. Repeat.

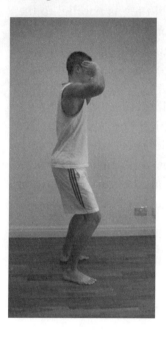 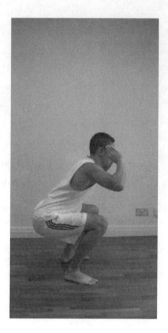 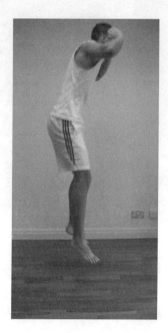

The Invisible Chair

This movement develops the thighs, and gluteal muscles. Unlike many other exercises, this one requires that you remain stationary in a stress position. You should aim to hold the position for as long as possible.

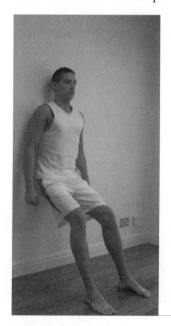 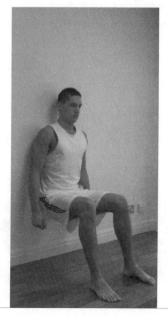

1.   Stand leaning with your back flat against a wall and your knees slightly bent. Your feet should be a little farther than shoulder width apart. Your toes should be pointing out slightly.
2.   Slowly lower your body down so that the tops of your thighs are parallel to the floor. Safety Note: Avoid lowering the body so far that your knees extend over your toes as this puts excessive strain on the knee joints.

3. This is a great exercise for ensuring continuous tension. Hold in the stress position until the muscles are fatigued and then slowly return back to the starting position.

Alternating Lunges

This is an explosive exercise for development of the thighs and gluteal muscles.

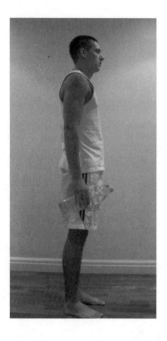 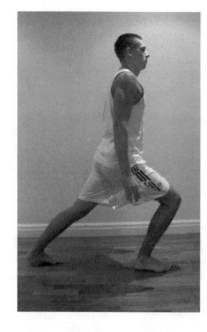

1. Adopt a standing position. Feet shoulder-width apart.
2. Take a large stride forward with your right foot. Firmly plant that foot on the floor and bend the knee until the thigh of your right leg is parallel to the floor. Safety Note: Ensure that your knee never extends beyond your foot, as this will place excessive strain on the knee joints.
3. At this point, your left leg should be extended behind you, knee slightly bent with your left heel raised above the floor. Explosively, push with your right leg back into the starting position. Repeat with your left leg.

Leg Extension with Briefcase

This is an isolation exercise, focusing on the quadriceps and is to be performed using a briefcase or similar item.

1. Sit on a chair or at the end of a bench with your legs slightly parted. Support the briefcase on your shins by pointing your toes upwards.
2. Raise the legs simultaneously until the legs are straight out in front of you. Flex the quadriceps at the top of the movement and then lower your legs back again.
3. To ensure continuous tension, do not lower your feet all the way back to the bottom. Keep your feet about 8 inches away from the floor.

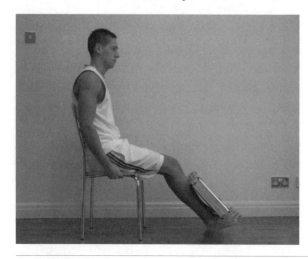 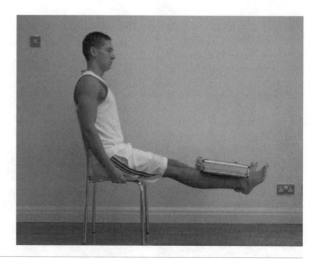

Standing Single-Leg Calf Raise

This exercise uses only your own bodyweight and focuses very well on the calf muscles. All you need is a staircase. (If you live in a bungalow, you may use a large, sturdy book!)

1. Stand on the first step of your staircase, holding the handrail for support. Stand on your left leg, positioning your foot so that only the balls of your feet and your toes are touching the step. The midsection and heel of your foot should be hanging over the edge of the step. Cross your right foot behind your left ankle.
2. Slowly rise all the way up onto your tiptoes, pause for a moment and then lower back down again. Vince claims for this exercise that it is important to get a good stretch on the calves so when you lower back down again, go as low as possible. Repeat.
3. Change legs and repeat until fatigued.

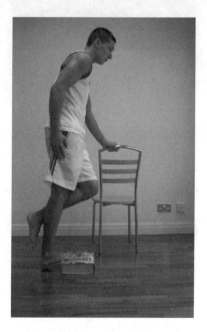 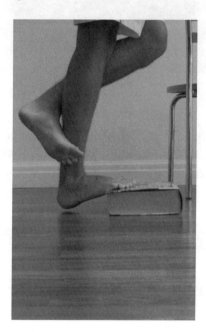 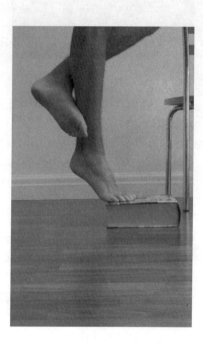

Donkey Calf Raise

This is another exercise intended to strengthen the muscles in the calves. This exercise can be performed either using the staircase again or by using a large book and a bench.

1. Stand on the book (or first step) with both feet together, positioned in the same way as in the previous exercise. Extend your arms out and lean on the bench in front of you (or third or fourth step). Keep your knees slightly bent.
2. Slowly lift up onto your tiptoes. Hold for a second, and then slowly lower your heels as far as they will go.

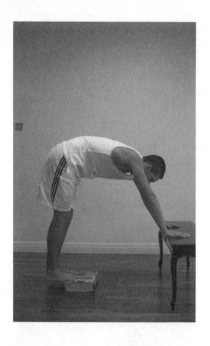
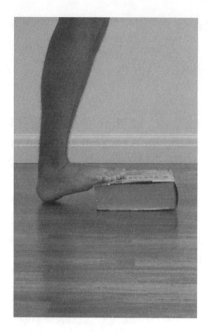
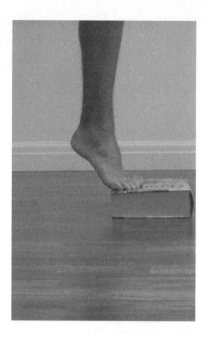

Suggested Leg Routines

To ensure continuous improvement, it's important to keep changing the routine so that your body doesn't grow accustomed to carrying out the same routine. We will ensure constant change by using different combinations of exercises and also by utilising the various core techniques of the Vince Graham System (supersets, super slow, explosive power and so on).

Please note that prior to starting the workout, it is advisable to spend a few minutes stretching or warming up by jogging on the spot or going for a brisk walk.

Week One: The Superset Program

A great method that Vince incorporates into his system is a technique used by bodybuilders known as the 'Superset'. For more information on this, you can refer back to the section on supersets in Chapter 2.

As you already are aware, to increase the effectiveness of a compound movement, we must use an isolation exercise to pre-exhaust the target muscle group. In this instance, we will be using the briefcase leg extension as a pre-exhaustion exercise for the quadriceps before performing the compound movements for the thighs.

The compound movements we will be using are single leg squats and alternating lunges. I chose this combination of compound movements because the single leg squat is a highly effective exercise for the quadriceps, hamstrings and glutes, as is the alternating lunge. The alternating lunge however adds variety due to it being an explosive power movement.

You will be required to perform each exercise to failure (until your final repetition results in failure – you just can't lift it). Then, as soon as you fail to perform the final repetition on the first exercise, you must progress immediately to the second exercise and perform the exercise to failure. And so on until you have completed the four exercises in the superset.

Upon completion of the superset, you will be allowed a short amount of time to rest (30-60 seconds) before commencing the superset for a second time. You must continue with the process until you have completed 7 minutes of activity. And here's the bad news – you are not allowed to count the rest period (30-60 seconds) between supersets as part of the total 7 minutes.

Listed below is the order in which you must completed the exercises for the leg superset:

1. Leg Extensions with Briefcase, performed to failure.
2. Alternating Lunges, performed to failure.
3. Leg Extensions with Briefcase, performed to failure.
4. Single Leg Squats, performed to failure.

*IMPORTANT NOTE: Remember, you must not rest between performing the different exercises listed above. You can only rest upon completion of these exercises for a period of 30 to 60 seconds before repeating the superset.

Week Two: The Explosive Power Program

The explosive power programme will really help to develop strength by over emphasising the positive portion of the exercise. The positive portion should be performed with speed and power and the negative portion performed at normal speed.

With this routine, the Alternating Lunge and Squat Jump are naturally performed in an explosive fashion, hence their inclusion in this routine. The Donkey calf raise should be included, although you may find it difficult to perform it explosively.

1. Perform Alternating Lunges for 2 minutes.
2. Perform Donkey Calf Raises for 2 minutes.
3. Perform the Squat Jump for 2 minutes.
4. Perform Alternating Lunges for 1 minute.

Week Three: The Negatives Programme

When performing exercises using the negatives method, it is important to perform the negative portion of the exercise slowly but the positive portion at the normal speed.

1. Perform the Standing Squat emphasising the negative portion for 2 minutes.
2. Perform the Standing Single Leg Calf Raise emphasising the negative portion for 2 minutes.
3. Perform the Invisible chair for 1 minute.
4. Perform the Leg Extension with Briefcase for 2 minutes emphasising the negative portion.

Week 4: The Super-Slow Programme

The super-slow method is very difficult and involves performing each repetition for roughly ten seconds. Five seconds for the positive and five seconds for the negative portion of the exercise. Super slow movements are highly effective because the duration of the exercise ensures that all the muscle fibres are fully engaged, resulting in 'peak contraction'.

1. Perform the Standing Squat for 1 minute.
2. Perform Leg Extension with Briefcase for 1 minute.
3. Perform Donkey Calf Raises for 1 minute.
4. Perform the Invisible Chair for 1 minute.
5. Perform Alternating Lunges for 1 minute.
6. Perform Single Leg Calf Raises for 2 minutes (1 minute per leg).

Chapter Nine
Friday: Arms Workout

Warming Up

I know of no specific stretching or warm-up exercises that concentrate on the muscles in the upper arms (the biceps and triceps). However, it is important that we do something prior to training these muscles that will prepare them for the workout ahead. To warm up the muscles, I have improvised a short series of movements. This warm up is merely a combination of light resistance exercises and muscle flexing to gently break the muscles in for more intense activity that will follow. Follow these steps to ensure your arms are correctly warmed up:

1. Raise your right arm up to shoulder level and perform the ever-popular biceps pose by flexing the biceps muscle. If you struggle to tense the muscle, keep the elbow bent at about 90 degrees and imagine trying to stop somebody straightening out your arm. You will know when you are tensing the biceps correctly as they will feel firmer as they are flexed. Repeat the same exercise with the left arm. Perform 2-3 repetitions with each arm, holding each repetition for around 10 seconds.
2. Extend your right arm down at your side. Try to extend the arm as far as possible, so that it could not be straighter. As you do this, try to tense the triceps in the back of your arm. You will know that you are tensing the muscles correctly if the triceps muscles feel firmer when you flex them. Repeat the same exercise with your left arm. Perform 2-3 repetitions with each arm, holding each repetition for around 10 seconds.
3. Pick up 2, light, water-filled bottles (perhaps 1 litre), one in each hand. In a standing position, with your palms facing forwards, simultaneously curl the bottles up towards your torso, whilst keeping your elbows stationary and tucked in at your sides. Perform 15 repetitions.
4. Using one of the lightweight bottles you used in the previous exercise, adopt a standing position. Grasp the bottle in both hands above the head with both arms straight, pointing to the ceiling. Keeping your elbows stationary, in the same position, bend at your elbows, lowering the bottle down behind your head. At this point, your elbows should be fully bent and pointing towards the ceiling. When you have lowered the bottle to head level, press the bottle back up to starting position. Repeat for 15 repetitions.

By performing light resistance exercises, and muscle tensing, you are able to warm up the muscles without performing specific stretching exercises. However, where possible, it is better to perform stretching movements as they are able to properly activate the muscle fibres and also, many people believe that the stretching exercises are effective in actually shaping and toning the muscles. Hence why many celebrities such as Brad Pitt and Madonna practice yoga movements in their spare time.

The Arms Workout

Water Bottle Alternating Curls

This exercise focuses on the biceps muscles in the upper arms.

1. Stand straight with your feet shoulder-width apart and your knees slightly bent. Hold a 2 litre water-filled bottle in each hand, with your arms fully extended at your sides and your palms facing in.
2. Slowly curl your left arm up towards your shoulders, keeping your upper arm and elbow stationary. As you curl the bottle, rotate your wrist through 90 degrees so that at the top of the movement, your palm is facing towards your chest. Slowly lower the bottle back to starting position and repeat with the right arm.
3. To ensure continuous tension, when you lower the bottle back down again, do not fully extend the arm at the bottom. Repeat until fatigued.

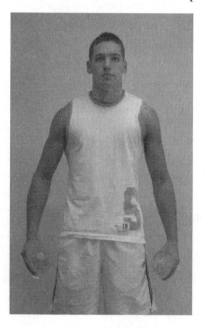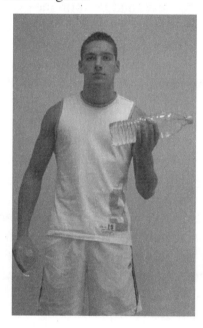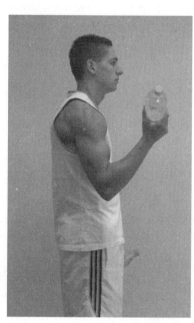

Water Bottle Concentration Curl

This exercise is a typical example of an isolation exercise. Hence its name... 'The concentration curl' and focuses almost entirely on the biceps.

1. Sit in a chair or at the end of a bench or bed with your feet planted firmly on the floor, a little farther than shoulder width apart. Hold a water bottle in your right hand, your palm facing your left leg. Rest your right elbow against your right thigh and allow your arm to fully extend, hanging down. With your left hand on your left thigh, bend forwards slightly, keeping your back straight.
2. Slowly curl the water bottle up towards your shoulder, keeping your upper arm stationary, and your elbow in contact with your thigh. Hold for a second at the top, before lowering the weight. Repeat until fatigued and then repeat using your other left arm.
3. To maintain continuous tension, when you lower the bottle back down to the bottom, ensure your elbow remains slightly bent to eliminate the rest period at the bottom portion of the exercise.

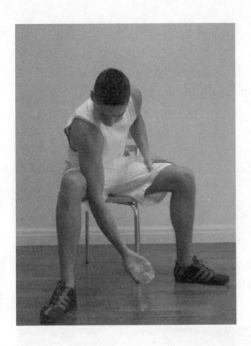 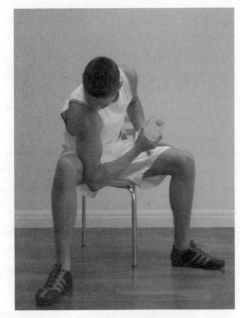

Water Bottle Hammer Curls

This exercise focuses on the outer portion of the biceps and also works the muscles in the forearms.

1. Stand straight with your feet shoulder-width apart and your knees slightly bent. Hold a 2 litre water-filled bottle in each hand, with your arms fully extended at your sides and your palms facing in.
2. Slowly curl both your arms up towards your shoulders, keeping your upper arms and elbows stationary. Do not rotate the wrists. At the top of the movement, your palms should be facing on another. Slowly lower the bottles back to starting position and repeat.
3. To ensure continuous tension, when you lower the bottles back down again, do not fully extend the arms at the bottom. Repeat until fatigued.

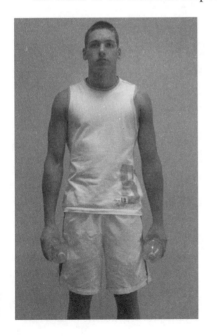 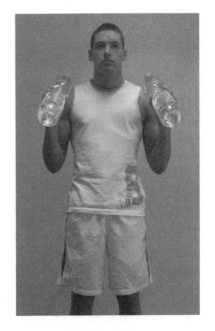 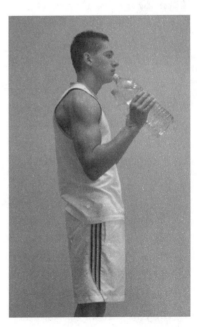

Curl Grip Chins

The chin is a very versatile exercise. Chinning movements exercise both the back muscles and the biceps. You should be aware that close grip movements focus more on the biceps and wider grip movements focus more on the back. Wider grip movements are more difficult because the biceps are less able to help the back muscles perform the exercise.

1. Adopt a position similar to previous chinning movements, but this time, grasp the bar with an underhand grip (palms facing towards you), with your hands narrower than shoulder width apart.
2. Slowly pull yourself up until your chin is level with the bar. Pause for a moment and then lower yourself back again.
3. In previous chinning movements, Vince recommended you ensure a good stretch at the bottom by allowing yourself to hang for a moment. As this exercise is for biceps and not the upper back, this principle does not apply. Ensure continuous tension by not fully extending the arms at the bottom of the movement. Repeat.

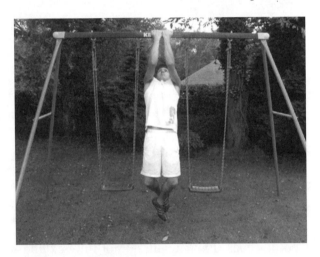 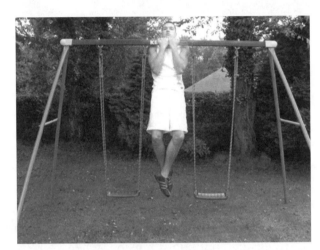

The Triceps Press-up

This variation of the classic exercise emphasises the triceps. It should be noted that when performing a press-up, a wider grip focuses on the pectorals and a really close grip focuses on the triceps. In the section on chest, I included a press-up exercise to emphasise the inner chest with hands placed at slightly closer than shoulder-width apart. The triceps press-up is similar but should be performed with the hands actually touching one another.

1. Adopt the classic press-up position with your back and legs forming a straight line. Adopt a hand position whereby your hands are touching. Vince performs this exercise with his hands in a position such that his forefingers and thumbs are in contact, forming a diamond shaped area of space between the hands. This will make the exercise more comfortable.
2. Slowly lower the body as close to the floor as possible. You will not be able to go as low as with the classic press-up because your hands and arms will get in the way. Pause for a moment at the bottom before raising your body back up again.
3. This is a difficult exercise and you may wish to perform it 'easy style', supporting your weight on your knees rather than the balls of your feet. Even in 'easy style', you should adopt a position whereby your upper legs and back form a straight line.
4. To maintain continuous tension, refrain from over-extending the arms at the top of the movement.

CHAPTER 9   The Vince Graham 7 Minute A Day Miracle Body Sculpting Programme

62

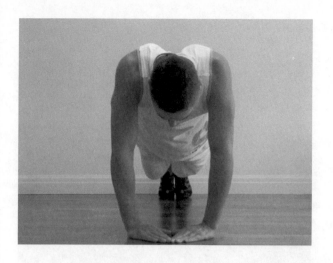 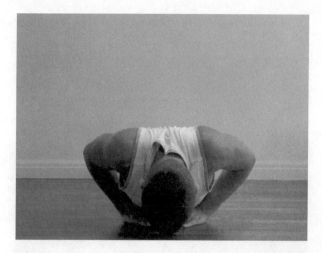

Water Bottle French Press Behind The Neck

This exercise works the triceps muscles and requires one two-litre or four-litre bottle filled with water.

1. Grip the bottle at each end and lift it over your head. Keep your upper arms stationary either

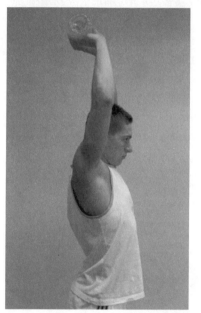 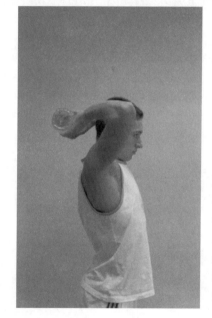

side of your head.
2. Slowly lower the bottle down behind your head until your arms are at an angle of ninety degrees. At this point, your elbows should be pointing towards the ceiling. Then slowly press the weight back to the starting position. You should keep your upper arms and elbows stationary throughout the exercise.
3. Ensure constant tension in this exercise by not fully extending the arms at the top of the movement.

Triceps Water Bottle Kickback

This exercise is a great movement for hitting the triceps.

1. Holding a water-filled bottle in your right hand, kneel on a bench with your left knee, supporting your balance by placing your left hand on the bench as well. Keep your right foot planted on the ground, with your back straight and parallel to the floor. Your right arm should be bent at 90 degrees with your right forearm perpendicular to the floor.
2. Slowly straighten out your arm, lifting the bottle behind your body until your right arm is straight and pointing behind you. Pause for a moment before lowering the arm to the starting position. Ensure continuous tension by not allowing the arm to return back to a position perpendicular to the floor.

3. Repeat until fatigued and then repeat using the right arm.

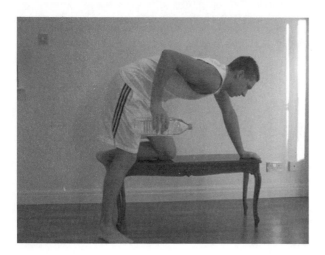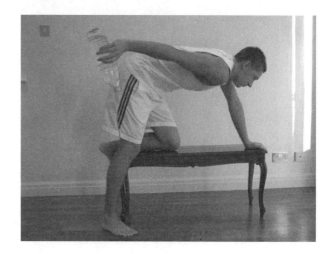

Lying Water Bottle Triceps Extension

This move is another great exercise for the triceps. Safety Note: Take care not to drop the bottle as this could result in facial injury.

1. Lie on your back on a bench. Extend your arms out to hold a water bottle with both hands above your head. Your elbows should not be locked out to ensure continuous tension.
2. Keep your upper arms and elbows stationary. Your elbows should point towards the ceiling. Slowly bend at your elbows and lower the weight down behind your head. Pause for a moment before pressing the weight back up to the starting position. Repeat until fatigued.

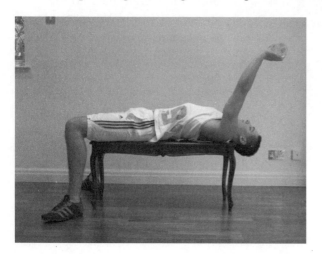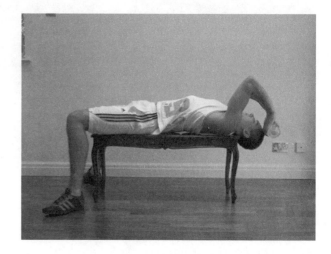

Suggested Arm Routines

To ensure continuous improvement, it is important to keep changing the routine so that the body does not grow accustomed to carrying out the same routine. We will ensure constant change by using different combinations of exercises and also by utilising the various core techniques of the Vince Graham System (supersets, super slow, explosive power and so on).

Please note that prior to starting the workout, it is advisable to spend a few minutes stretching or even warming up by jogging on the spot or going for a brisk walk.

Week One: The Superset Program

A great method that Vince incorporates into his system is a technique used by bodybuilders known as the 'Superset'. For more information on this, you can refer back to the section on supersets in Chapter 2.

For this superset, we will be using the pre-exhaustion principle to increase the effectiveness of the Curl Grip Chins and Triceps Press-up movements, as these are compound movements. To achieve this, we must partially tire (pre-exhaust) the biceps and triceps respectively before performing the compound techniques. Performing isolation exercises such as Water Bottle Concentration Curls (for biceps) and Water Bottle Triceps Kickbacks can achieve this.

You will be required to perform each exercise to failure (until your final repetition results in failure – you just can't lift it). Then, as soon as you fail to perform the final repetition on the first exercise, you must progress immediately to the second exercise and perform the exercise to failure. And so on until you have completed the four exercises in the superset.

Upon completion of the superset, you will be allowed a short amount of time to rest (30-60 seconds) before commencing the superset for a second time. You must continue with the process until you have completed 7 minutes of activity. And here's the bad news – you are not allowed to count the rest period (30-60 seconds) between supersets as part of the total 7 minutes.

Listed below is the order in which you must complete the exercises for the arms superset. Although the upper arms are comprised of two muscle groups, we can still train them at the same time. I have included the isolation exercises first, followed by two compound movements. The beauty of this superset is that when you train the triceps, the biceps can rest and vice versa, but we still get the benefits of pre-exhaustion. So here goes...

1. Water Bottle Concentration Curls (Both arms), performed to failure.
2. Lying Water Bottle Triceps Extensions, performed to failure.
3. Curl Grip Chins, performed to failure.
4. Close Grip Triceps Press-ups, performed to failure.

*IMPORTANT NOTE: Remember, you must not rest between performing the different exercises listed above. You can only rest upon completion of these exercises for a period of 30 to 60 seconds before repeating the superset.

Week Two: The Explosive Power Program

The explosive power programme will really help to develop strength by over emphasising the positive portion of the exercise. The positive portion should be performed with speed and power and the negative portion performed at normal speed.

1. Perform the Water Bottle Alternating Curls for 2 minutes.
2. Perform Water Bottle Hammer Curls for 2 minutes.
3. Perform the Water Bottle French Press Behind the Neck for 2 minutes.
4. Perform the Triceps Press-Up for 1 minute.

Week Three: The Negatives Programme

When performing exercises using the negative method, it is important to perform the negative portion of the exercise slowly but the positive portion at the normal speed.

1. Perform the Curl Grip Chins, emphasising the negative portion for 1 minute.
2. Perform Water Bottle Hammer Curls emphasising the negative portion for 2 minutes.
3. Perform Water Bottle Triceps Kickbacks emphasising the negative portion for 2 minute (1 minute per arm).
4. Perform the Lying Water Bottle Triceps Extension for 2 minutes emphasising the negative portion.

Week 4: The Super-Slow Programme

The super-slow method is very difficult and involves performing each repetition for roughly ten seconds. Five seconds for the positive and five seconds for the negative portion of the exercise. Super slow movements are highly effective because the duration of the exercise ensures that all the muscle fibres are fully engaged, resulting in 'peak contraction'.

1. Perform Water Bottle Alternating Curls for 1 minute.
2. Perform Water Bottle Hammer Curls for 1 minute.
3. Perform Water Bottle Concentration Curls for 2 minutes (1 minute per arm).
4. Perform the Water Bottle French Press Behind the Neck for 1 minute.
5. Perform the Lying Water Bottle Triceps Extension for 2 minutes.

CHAPTER TEN
Saturday: Abdominals

Everybody wants great abs. The abdominals are the single best indicator of the quality of an individual's physique. As well as being highly desirable to the opposite sex, the abdominals play an important role in maintaining good posture and protecting the vital organs.

The problem here is that everybody has their own ideas about how to carve out that 'six-pack' and one look at the people around you would suggest that most are mistaken. So why... you ask, are so many people sweating away for hours and not achieving the results that they deserve? The answer to this is simple...misinformation.

Myths And Misinformation

Because flat, 'washboard' abdominals are seen as the most highly desired attribute in any physique, every man and his dog has tried to sell you some new-fangled 'thingy' that will transform you from Rik Waller to David Beckham in only 6 weeks!

You shouldn't really need telling that these scams and gadgets don't work. Hollywood actor, bodybuilder and author, Steve Reeves had great abdominals in the 1940s and 1950s and this was long before the marketers began their work. If you walk through that pasture full of bulls, be prepared for what you might step in.

Many people believe that the best way to achieve great abs is to do endless amounts of sit-ups every day, in an effort to develop the muscles and burn the fat between those muscles. If you are one of these believers, I've got news for you...

Performing sit-ups for hours on end will actually make you look fatter! Yes, that's right. You see everybody has got a six-pack. It's just that you will have no chance of seeing it if it's hidden beneath an inch of lard. If you insist on performing gut-busting abdominal routines, you will only succeed in making the abdominals larger, which will merely push the fat out farther. Making your abdomen protrude will completely ruin your chances of achieving that slim waistline and V shaped appearance.

One commonly held myth is that performing abdominal exercises will burn the fat between the muscles in a process referred to as spot-reducing.

The idea of spot-reducing is to target fat-loss in certain areas of the body with specific exercises for that part of the body. So if you have fat on your abdomen, so the theory goes, you need to do lots of abdominal exercises to attack the fat. Guess what? .... This theory is complete nonsense.

It is scientifically impossible to target fat loss to one specific area of the body. In order to lose fat in one place, you have got to lose fat everywhere. And the best way to do this is simply to perform more calorie burning cardiovascular exercise.

The principle is simple. To burn fat, you merely need to burn more calories than you consume. If you want those abs, concentrate on reducing the amount of carbohydrates in your diet, because if your body runs out of carbohydrates, it will turn to its fat stores for energy. For more information on nutrition, refer back to chapter 3.

Some people achieve the six-pack look by doing little or no abdominal training. For example, Denise Lewis the British Heptathlete possesses textbook abdominals and rarely performs abdominal exercises. The reason for her success is down to a combination of fat loss through exercise and good genetics. You see some people are lucky enough to have naturally well-shaped abdominal muscles. All these people have to do is simply burn the excess fat away to make them visible.

So Why Bother Training The Abs At All?

Well. To improve the appearance of the abdominal area, it is important to actually firm the muscles – not build them up. By performing the Vince Graham abdominal workout once per week, you can improve the appearance of your stomach simply by firming and shaping the muscles slightly. If you haven't got naturally well-shaped abdominals like Denise Lewis, performing Vince's workout once per week can help to improve their natural shape without making the muscles larger.

The common belief is that the sit-up is the best exercise for improving the abdominal muscles. Yet many people perform 50,100 or even 200 sit-ups every day and achieve very little. The truth is that the sit up…as it is usually performed…is not particularly effective. It doesn't focus on the important shape-enhancing muscles.

The Way Forward

Other exercises do the job so much better, and Vince has carefully handpicked the most effective abdominal exercises, for you to use in the workout. A study led by Peter Francis, Ph.D., at the bio-mechanics lab at San Diego State University put different abdominal exercises to the test and found that not all are created equal.

The traditional sit-up fell close to the bottom in a ranking of the ab exercises. What makes the traditional sit-up ineffective is that many people sit all the way up, relying on their hips and less on their abdominals, not only making the sit-up ineffective but also placing strain on the back.

The study also found that (surprise, surprise) despite the advertising hype, most abdominal exercise equipment tested, was no more effective or only marginally more effective, than a regular crunch you can do at no cost.

The study revealed that the most highly effective abdominal exercise was the Bicycle Manoeuvre – an exercise that you have probably never even heard of before! The Vince Graham system will show you how to correctly perform this wonder exercise as well as some other highly effective exercises to target different areas of the abdomen. No stretching or warming up is required for the abdominals so let's get started...

The Abdominal Workout

Bicycle Manoeuvre

This super-exercise for the abdominals was found to be 250% more effective than the sit-up in a study carried out at San Diego State University.

1. To do this exercise, you lie flat on the floor with your lower back pressed to the ground. Raise your buttocks up, off the floor.
2. Bring your knees up to about a 45-degree angle and slowly go through a bicycle pedal motion.
3. Breathe evenly throughout the exercise. Continue until fatigued.

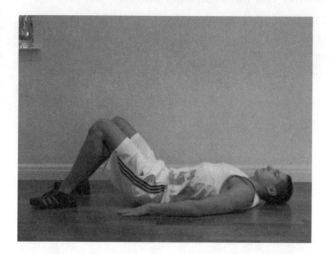 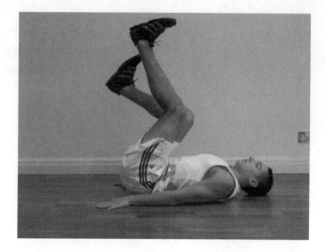

V-Sit Up

This exercise is a far more effective version of the regular sit-up, utilising the movement of the legs to increase the tension on the abdominals.

1. Lie flat on the floor, face-up with your arms crossed over your chest and your legs stretched out.
2. Simultaneously curl your torso upwards and bend your knees, bringing your thighs towards your body. Pause for a second before straightening the body again.
3. To ensure continuous tension, do not lie back down again. Instead, straighten the legs out and go back to a position where your legs and shoulders are suspended off the floor.

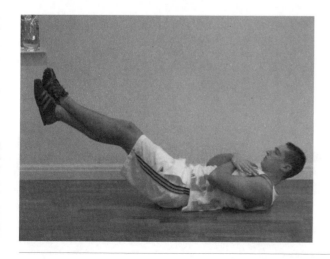 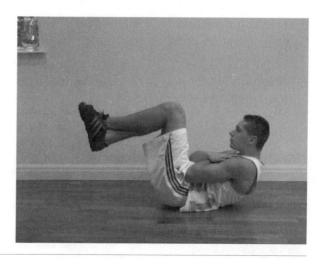

The Intensity Crunch

A crunch differs from a sit-up in that you do not bend your body at the hips. Your focus should be on raising the shoulders as high as possible off the floor, whilst keeping your lower back in contact with the floor. You must use only your abdominal muscles to achieve this.

1. Lay on your back with your feet braced against or under a stationary object. Your knees should be bent at 90 degrees. Cross your arms across your chest.
2. Begin a normal crunch movement by slowly raising your shoulders away from the ground. Remember to keep your lower back in contact with the floor to eliminate the hips from the movement.
3. When you reach your most intense contracted position you must put all your attention into the abdominal area tensing it as hard as possible for a count of 2.
4. Keeping your abs as tense as possible slowly return to a prone position. It should take you at least 3 seconds to reach a position, just inches away from the floor.
5. When you reach this position, keep maximum tension on the abs and repeat the motion.
6. Continue repetitions to failure.

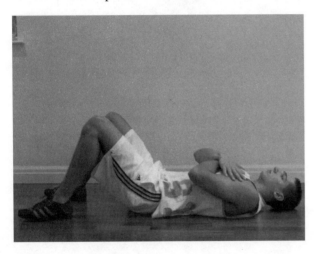 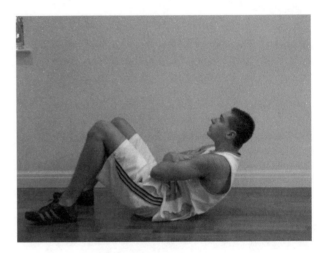

Isometric Tension

Isometric tension is a very versatile tool for training the abs and will enable you to perform abdominal exercises almost anywhere (whilst driving to work, or standing in a queue at the paper shop).

1. Stand straight up.
2. Concentrate as hard as you can on your abs.
3. Tense your abs as hard as possible. Put all your energy into tensing your abs.
4. Maintain the tension for a count of 6 and relax.
5. Immediately tense the abs again.
6. Continue this cycle until fatigued.

IMPORTANT NOTE: If performing isometrics in public, please ensure that you have full control over your facial expressions!

Abdominal Inching

This unusual and highly effective exercise is rarely used but is one of the few exercises that will focus on the lower abdominals.

1. Sit on the floor, legs together, stretched out in front of you. Keep your back erect and clasp your hands across your chest.
2. Using the power of your abs and hips try to inch across the floor for a distance of 10 feet. Do not bend your knees or get your back or arms into the movement.
3. Using your lower abs move your right hip and then your left hip and inch. Continue until you reached 10 feet or cannot move further.
4. Rest 90 seconds and repeat this movement backwards to your starting spot.
5. After you have mastered this exercise place a weight in your lap for greater resistance.

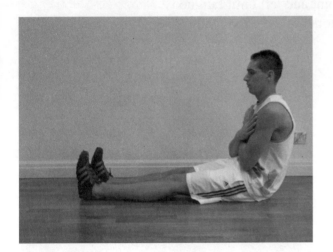 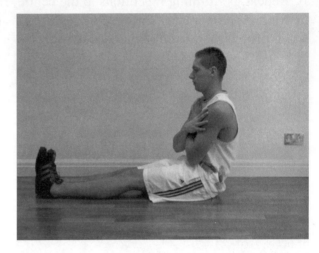

End of Bench Leg-Raises

This is also a lower abdominal exercise, however the upper abdominals are also recruited slightly.

1. Lie flat on your back on a normal exercise bench with your hips at the lower end.
2. Hold the upper end of the bench with your hands.
3. Keeping your legs together, bend them up towards your chest.
4. Slowly extend your legs and straighten your knees until your body is perfectly straight with your legs hanging over the end of the bench.
5. Pause for a moment and then slowly bend at the knees and bring your legs back up to the starting position.
6. Repeat until fatigued.

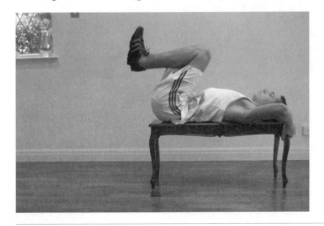 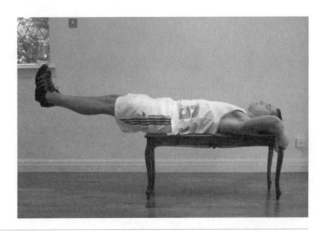

The Twist-up

This is a variation of the Sit-Up. Twisting alternatively from side to side will additionally involve the intercostals between the ribs as well as the obliques.

1. Lie on your back on the floor and hook your toes under a heavy piece of furniture. Bend your knee comfortably and keep them bent for the duration of the movement. This helps to relieve back strain.
2. Place your hands behind your head and lock your fingers together.
3. Curl your torso upwards of the floor until it is at an angle of around 45 degrees. Hold the upright position for a second and reverse the movement slowly until reaching the starting point.
4. Perform a second repetition. However, this time, twist to the right as you raise yourself.
5. Perform a third repetition twisting to the left.
6. Repeat, performing repetitions to the centre, right and left until fatigued.
7. Maintain continuous tension by keeping your torso off the floor and by not going farther than 45 degrees at the top of the movement.

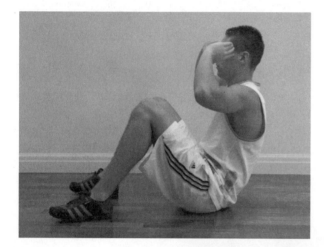
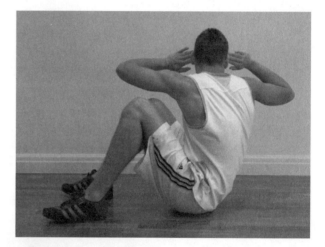
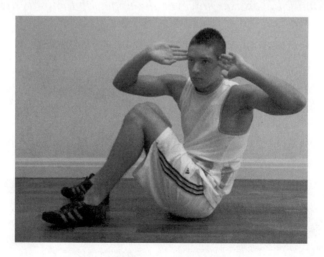

Water Bottle Side Bends

This exercise focuses the tension on the obliques.

1. Stand up straight and hold a two-litre bottle in each hand.
2. Bend sideways holding your pelvis firmly.
3. When you reach a point where you cannot bend further, inhale, hold your breath and raise yourself back to the erect starting position exhaling when you reach the vertical position.
4. Repeat this movement, this time bending to the opposite side. Repeat until fatigued.

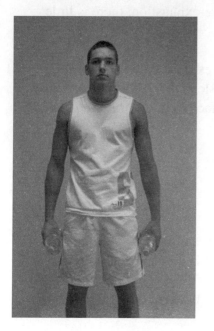
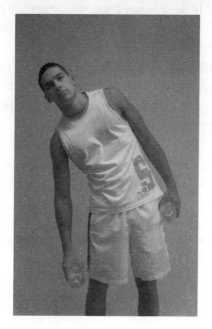
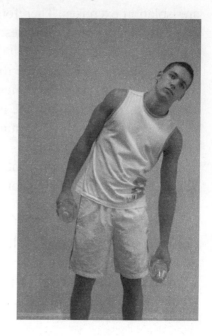

Broomstick Twists

A good exercise for the obliques that can also be used as a calorie burning movement. You will require a broomstick.

1. Hold a broomstick in both hands, behind the neck, adopting a wide grip.

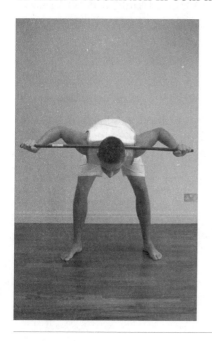
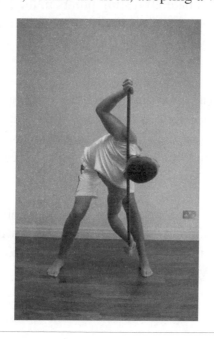
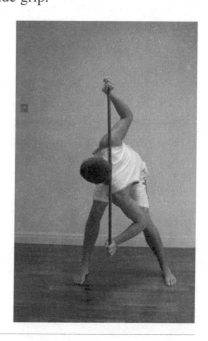

2. Bend at the waist until your torso is almost parallel to the floor.
3. Twist your body and touch your left foot with the right hand side of the broomstick. Then, immediately twist the other way to touch your right foot with the left hand side of the broomstick. Repeat for the required duration.

Suggested Abdominal Routines

The following workout routines will differ somewhat from the routines for the other body parts. There will not be a separate routine for Supersets because all exercises for the abdominal muscles are isolation exercises. Therefore, if we cannot take advantage of pre-exhaustion, there is little point in Super-setting exercises.

Neither will there be separate routines for negatives, super-slow, or explosive power. The reason for this is that that all abdominal exercises should be performed as slowly as possible in order to gain full recruitment of all the muscle fibres. There are three main factors in ensuring the effectiveness of an abdominal training programme:

1. The speed of the movement.
2. Ensuring continuous tension.
3. Performing the right exercises.

For most exercises, you should aim to perform the movement slowly and smoothly, using only the abdominals to control the movement. If performed correctly, you will feel a deep burning sensation in the muscles and the following day, the muscles will probably feel a little sore. Don't worry, this soreness will subside in a week or too as soon as the muscles in the abdomen have strengthened.

Exercises, which should be performed at a moderate speed, are Broomstick Twists and the Bicycle Manoeuvre. Isometrics are obviously performed from a stationary position. Abdominal Inching can be performed at any speed that feels comfortable as long as you are careful not to rush the movement, and ensure that the lower abdominals are doing all of the work.

The second factor contributing to success is ensuring continuous tension when performing the exercises. You should strive to eliminate all resting points in the movements. Doing this will make the exercises more difficult and you may need to rest more frequently, but the quality of the exercise will be greatly improved and you will notice improvements more quickly.

The final factor is to perform the most effective exercises. This is simple – the ones listed above are the best exercises so don't waste your time with other techniques. If a friend informs you of a new abdominal exercise, take a good look at them. If you think they might have a six-pack lurking beneath their sweatshirt, listen to what they have to say. If they look as though their abs are covered in 3 inches of lard, be polite but stick to the exercises in the Vince Graham System. Trust me. They work!

Listed below are a number of routines proposed by Vince that comprise of exercises that work well together. Each routine is made up of exercises that hit the lower abdominals, upper abdominals and obliques. Give each one a try to add some variety to your abdominal training. Remember, constant change is the key to the Vince Graham system.

Workout One:

1. Perform the Bicycle Manoeuvre for 3 minutes.
2. Perform Abdominal Inching for 2 minutes.
3. Perform the Twist-up for 2 minutes.

Workout Two:

1. Perform the V Sit-up for 3 minutes.
2. Perform End of Bench Leg Raises for 2 minutes.
3. Perform Water Bottle Side Bends for 2 minutes.

Workout Three:

1. Perform Isometric Tension for 1 minute.
2. Perform the Intensity Crunch for 2 minutes.
3. Perform End of Bench Leg Raises for 2 minutes.
4. Perform Broomstick Twists for 2 minutes.

Workout Four:

1. Perform Isometric Tension for 1 minute.
2. Perform the Intensity Crunch for 1 minute.
3. Perform the Bicycle Manoeuvre for 1 minute.
4. Perform Abdominal Inching for 1 minute.
5. Perform End of Bench Leg Raises for 1 minute.
6. Perform Water Bottle Side Bends for 1 minute.
7. Perform Broomstick Twists for 1 minute.

I just want to emphasise this again because it's so important…you will never have great looking abdominals until you remove the layer of fat which is covering them. Strong abdominal muscles act to pull in the fat so that you look slimmer in clothes, but when you remove your shirt, the truth will be revealed.

Imagine a great sculpture and then put it in bubble-wrap. Is anyone going to appreciate the intricacy of the carving? I rest my case.

CHAPTER ELEVEN
Nutrition

The Vince Graham 7 Minute A Day Body Sculpting Programme is not about dieting. It is about sculpting the perfect body. I don't want spend this chapter introducing you to yet another new diet programme that won't work. In fact, Vince specifically asked me not to include a diet section in the book.

Vince simply doesn't believe in diets. He's never been on a diet in his whole life. In his view, the nutritional key to transforming your body is not a short term diet...but rather a long term change in eating habits.

Dieting is never effective in the long-term. You see, when you diet, you will perhaps lose quite a lot of weight in the first week or so because your metabolism is still high from you eating out the entire contents of the fridge, and then going back for the sweepings up!.

After a week or two of comparative fasting, your body re-adjusts. Your diet has fooled it into thinking you are suffering a famine. As a response, your body slows down its metabolic rate and begins to push fats into storage in case they are needed.

When you go back to eating normally, having lost the desired half a stone, your slower metabolic rate results in you putting all the weight that you lost back on again, in a very short time.

Thus, the end result of the diet is simply a yo-yo effect on your weight. And this puts tremendous stress on your body, because when it comes to nutrition, your body thrives on regularity. It is therefore far better to simply eat more efficiently on a regular basis, than to eat poorly and then starve yourself.

In this chapter, I want to give you some guidelines for 'eating correctly' as Vince puts it. It's not a diet...it's just a series of ideas and principles for you to incorporate into your day to day eating habits. Some you'll adopt as part of your life, some you'll do when you can, and others you'll probably reject altogether. But if you at least do something, and do it regularly, you'll be head and shoulders above the world's dieters.

Macronutrients

Firstly, I'd like to talk a little about the three macronutrients. These are carbohydrates, proteins and fats. Some people believe fats to be a mortal enemy, others say fat is okay and it is carbohydrates that should be feared (cue Dr. Atkins!). The truth of the matter is that all three of the macronutrients are okay. In fact, not just okay – absolutely essential. We do not however, need too much of a good thing. The key to a healthy, toned body is moderation.

Carbohydrates

Carbohydrates provide us with the energy we need to go about performing our 7-minute workout.

To perform exercise, our muscles need glycogen for fuel. Glycogen is simply a form of stored energy and of the three macro-nutrients (carbohydrates, fat, protein), it is carbohydrate that is most readily converted to glycogen.

So carbohydrates are important for the creation of a lean, muscular physique. But don't get carried away and start reaching for that Mars bar just yet. Although we do need carbohydrates, we need the right kind of carbohydrates. As we have already touched on in previous chapters, simple carbohydrates such as those we find in sweet foods are digested too quickly for most of our daily energy requirements. This results in an energy overload and the body begins to push fats into storage. This is a bad thing.

It is much better to get most of your carbohydrate intake in the form of complex carbohydrates such as those found in brown rice, wholegrain bread, pasta and vegetables. Because generally complex carbohydrates are broken down more slowly, they provide a steady, sustained source of energy for a longer period of time.

Following intense exercise, the muscles become depleted of glycogen so the best time to consume simple carbohydrates from sugary foods is immediately after your workout. This will replace the depleted glycogen and prevent muscle catabolism (muscle breakdown). Again, don't go for the chocolate bars. Fruit juice is a much healthier option that will also provide your body with vitamins and nutrients.

How Many Carbs?

You can use the following formulas to determine the amount of carbohydrates you should optimally consume each day. For this example, I will be using a 175-pound male who consumes 3000 calories per day. I have also recommended that 60% of your daily calorific intake should come from carbohydrates. Obviously, if you weigh less and/or you are female, you should decrease the number of calories accordingly.

The Formula:

Daily X Recommended Carbohydrate Consumption = Calories From
Calories   Carbs per Day

Example:

3000 X 0.6 = 1800 calories from carbohydrates.

To determine how many grams of carbohydrates needed each day, divide the number of calories by 4 (there are 4 calories per gram of carbohydrate). So...

1800 / 4 = 450 grams per day.

Protein

Protein is an essential macronutrient for anybody trying to sculpt the perfect body. In order to shape and firm the muscles, our body needs amino acids. Amino acids are the building blocks of

CHAPTER 11   The Vince Graham 7 Minute A Day Miracle Body Sculpting Programme

78

protein and the building blocks of muscle. Basically, if we want to develop the muscles, we have to consume adequate amounts of protein.

If you think back to earlier chapters, where we talked about how to make the muscles respond, you will remember that to harden and tone the muscles, we must first damage the muscle fibres. Once the muscle fibres are damaged, our bodies use protein and amino acids to make the muscles stronger, firmer, and larger than before.

If we don't consume enough protein, our bodies will be unable to grow better muscles. So to maximise the results you get from the Vince Graham system, it is worth thinking about the way that you eat protein. The general rule is to consume about 1.5 grams of protein per kilo of body-weight. The following equation will help you work out your requirement:

1. Firstly, you need to divide your weight in pounds by 2.2 (the number of pounds per kilogram) to give you your weight in kilos.
2. Then multiply your weight in kilos by 1.5 (your daily requirement).

Example:

175 pounds divided by 2.2 = 79.5 kilos.

79.5 multiplied by 1.5 = 119.25 grams per day.

Fats

Fat is an essential nutrient and should not be treated as a poison that will ruin your body. Like most things that we eat, too little fat is bad for us, and so is too much fat. The key here is moderation. You should also realise that some fats are better than others.

Fats found in vegetable oils, plants, nuts and seeds are some of the best kinds of fats, supplying our bodies with essential nutrients known as essential fatty acids or EFAs.

EFAs are essential nutrients and are contained in almost every cell in our bodies, with a great abundance being in the brain. In fact, 20% of the dry weight of the brain is made up of EFAs. There are two EFAs known as Omega 3 and Omega 6. These can be found in fish oil, vegetable oil and certain plants and fruits such as avocado. Nuts, seeds and pulses are also known to contain high quantities of these essential nutrients.

The 'bad' fats you should be aware of are those contained in dairy products, and meat. These fats are often saturated and contain high amounts of cholesterol – the stuff that heart disease is made of. Again, the fats contained in plant foods are better as they are unsaturated and can actually help to lower cholesterol. Instead of a bacon sandwich, opt for foods such as peanut butter or olive oil.

If you don't mind counting calories and grams, here's a formula that will enable you to calculate your daily fat requirement. When it comes to fats though, concentrate on quality, not quantity. Try to make sure that most of your fats come from plant sources.

Formula:

Daily Calories   X   Recommended Fat Intake (20%) = Calories from fat.

Example:

3000   X   0.2 (20%) = 660

In order to determine how many grams of fat you should consume, you need to divide the number of calories from fat per day by the number of calories in a gram of fat (nine).

Example:

660 / 9 = 73 grams per day.

Micronutrients

Aside from protein, carbohydrates and fats, we must also keep our bodies regularly topped up with plenty of vitamins and minerals. Although it is possible to derive an abundance of these nutrients from our daily food intake, nobody has the perfect diet all the time, and it may be a good idea to supplement your body with a multimineral-multivitamin product.

Listed below are a number of key vitamins and minerals that are needed to keep the body in tip-top condition and also where they can be found.

Vitamin A – Important for eyesight, skin and maintaining the mucus membranes in the nose and throat. Found in eggs, liver, milk, carrots, and spinach.

Vitamin B – (12 vitamins on total). Has a role in the nervous system and Complex   digestive system. Found in green vegetables, fruit, whole grains, eggs, and poultry.

Vitamin C – Plays an important role in immunity. Found in citrus fruits, and vegetables.

Vitamin D – Needed for strong teeth and bones due to increasing the absorption of calcium. Mostly from sunlight.

Vitamin E – Needed for proper functioning of the respiratory and reproductive systems. Found in vegetable oils, eggs, leafy vegetables and wheat germ.

Important minerals include: Calcium, chromium, magnesium, manganese and phosphorous. Obviously, calcium is needed for strong bones and teeth and is found in abundance in dairy produce. As for the others, if you eat plenty of fruit and vegetables, you can't go far wrong.

Now that you have calculated the amounts of protein, fat and carbohydrates you should be consuming each day, you will most likely want to know which foods contain what. To help get you started, I have included a list of 125 great 'hard-body' foods, complete with how many grams of each macronutrient you are likely to find in each as well as the number of calories. So here goes...

MEAT/FISH/POULTRY

FOOD	CAL	PRO (G)	CARB (G)	FAT (G)
Salmon (wild)	182	25	0	8
Back bacon, grilled, 2 slices	87	11	1	4
Canned light tuna	116	26	0	1
Canned white tuna	128	24	0	3
Chicken breast, skinless	160	31	0	4
Chicken drumstick, 1 skinless	76	12	0	3
Chicken thigh, 1 skinless	108	14	0	6
Cod	105	23	0	1
Crab	97	19	0	2
Roast beef, 1 oz. sliced	50	8	2	1
Extra-lean minced beef	171	26	0	7
Halibut	140	27	0	3
Ham, sliced, extra-lean	131	20	1	5
Lamb, choice, leg	205	22	0	12
Pork loin	164	28	0	5
Scallops	88	17	3	1
Shrimp 5 oz.	99	21	0	0
Silverside	175	28	0	6
Sirloin (grilled)	206	30	0	9
Topside (grilled)	176	32	0	5
Tuna, fresh	184	30	0	6
Turkey breast, skinless	135	30	0	0
Venison, tenderloin, grilled	149	30	0	2

Serving size is 3.5 oz., trimmed of all visible fat, roasted, unless otherwise noted

GRAINS/BREADS/PASTA

FOOD	CAL	PRO (G)	CARB (G)	FAT (G)
Barley, pearl, 1 c cooked	193	4	44	1
Brown rice, 1 c cooked	217	5	45	2
Corn tortilla, 1	58	2	12	1
Couscous, 1 c cooked	176	6	37	tr
Crumpet, 1	134	4	26	1
Flour tortilla, 8"	146	4	25	3
Macaroni, 1 c cooked	197	7	40	1
Oatmeal, 1 c cooked	142	6	25	2
Plain bagel, I small (3")	190	7	37	1
Spaghetti, 1 c cooked	197	7	40	1
Wheatgerm, 2 Tbsp.	52	4	8	1
White rice, 1 c cooked	205	4	45	tr
Wholegrain cereal, Total, 3/4 c	97	2	23	1
Wholemeal bread, I slice	73	3	13	1
Wholegrain crackers, 5	90	2	14	3

Wholemeal pitta, 1	170	6	35	2
Wild rice, 1 c cooked	166	7	35	1

FRUIT

FOOD	CAL	PRO (G)	CARB (G)	FAT (G)
Apple, 1 medium	72	tr	19	tr
Apricots, 3	50	2	12	tr
Avocado, 1/4	80	1	4	7
Banana, 1 medium	105	1	30	tr
Blueberries, I c	83	1	21	tr
Melon, 1 c	54	1	13	tr
Cherries, tart, 1 c pitted	78	2	19	tr
Grapefruit, 1/2 medium	41	1	10	tr
Grape juice, 1/2 c	77	tr	19	tr
Grapes, 1 c seedless	110	1	29	tr
Mango, 1 c cubes	107	1	28	tr
Nectarine, 1 medium	60	1	14	tr
Orange, 1 navel	69	1	18	tr
Orange juice, 1 c	112	2	26	tr
Peach, 1 medium	38	1	9	tr
Pear, 1 medium	96	1	26	tr
Pineapple, 1 c cubes	74	1	20	tr
Plum, 1	30	tr	8	tr
Raisins, 1/4 c (not packed)	108	1	29	tr
Raspberries, 1 c	64	2	15	1
Strawberries, 1 c	49	1	12	tr
Watermelon, 1 c cubes	46	1	12	tr

VEGETABLES

FOOD	CAL	PRO (G)	CARB (G)	FAT (G)
Artichoke, 1 medium	60	4	13	tr
Asparagus, 4 large spears	16	2	3	tr
Aubergine, 1/2 c cubed	10	tr	2	tr
Beetroot, 1 c sliced, cooked	75	3	17	tr
Broccoli florets, 1 c raw	25	2	4	tr
Brussels sprouts, 1c cooked	56	4	11	1
Butternut squash, 1c cubes,	82	2	22	tr
Cabbage, 1 c shredded	17	1	4	tr
Carrot, 1 large	30	1	7	tr
Cauliflower, 1 c	25	2	5	tr
Chinese cabbage, 1 c	20	3	3	tr
Corn, 1/2 c kernels	66	3	15	1
Courgette, 1 c chopped	20	2	4	tr
Cucumber, I c sliced	16	1	4	tr
Garlic, 1 clove	5	tr	1	tr

Food	CAL	PRO	CARB	FAT
Green beans, 1/2 c	17	1	4	tr
Green peas, 1/2 c raw	59	4	11	tr
Kale, 1 c chopped, cooked	36	3	7	1
Mushrooms, 1 c sliced	15	2	2	tr
Onion, 1/2 c chopped	33	1	8	tr
Pepper (green), 1 c chopped	30	1	7	tr
Potato, 1 med'm (6oz),baked	161	4	37	tr
Pumpkin, 1c fresh,, mashed	49	2	12	tr
Romaine lettuce, 1 c shredded	10	1	2	tr
Spinach, 1 c	7	1	1	tr
Tomato, 1 large	33	2	7	tr
Tomato juice, 1 c	41	2	10	tr
Tomato sauce, 1/2 c	39	2	9	tr

DAIRY/EGG PRODUCTS

FOOD	CAL	PRO (G)	CARB (G)	FAT (G)
Egg, large, 1 whole raw	74	6	tr	5
Egg substitute, 1/4 c liquid	53	8	tr	2
Egg white, 1 large raw	16	4	tr	tr
Low-fat buttermilk, 1 c	98	8	12	2
Low-fat cheddar cheese, 1 oz.	49	7	1	2
Low-fat cottage cheese, 1/2 c	81	14	3	1
Ricotta cheese, 1/2 c	171	14	6	10
Plain fat-free yogurt, 8 oz.	127	13	17	tr
Skimmed milk, 1 c	86	8	12	tr
Swiss cheese, low-fat, 1 oz.	50	8	1	1

LEGUMES

FOOD	CAL	PRO (G)	CARB (G)	FAT (G)
Baby lima beans, 1/2 c cooked	115	7	21	tr
Black beans, 1/2 c cooked	11	48	20	1
Chickpeas, 1/2 c cooked	134	7	23	2
Kidney beans, 1/2 c cooked	112	8	20	tr
Lentils, 1/2 c cooked	11	59	20	tr
Raw firm tofu, 3 1/2 oz.	145	16	4	9
Soya beans, 1/2 c cooked	127	11	10	6
Split peas, 1/2 c cooked	116	8	21	tr

NUTS/SEEDS/OILS

FOOD	CAL	PRO (G)	CARB (G)	FAT (G)
Almonds, 1 oz.	164	6	6	14
Almond butter, 2 Tbsp.	203	5	7	19
Olive oil, 1 Tbsp.	119	0	0	14
Peanut butter, 2 Tbsp.smooth	192	8	6	17
Peanuts, 1 oz. dry roasted	166	7	6	14
Walnuts, 1 oz.	185	4	4	19

(Standard Cup Measurement/1 cup = 250ml),(Nutritional values per serving will vary depending upon selectedbrands)

Calories And Weight: How Much Should You Eat?

The following tables indicate what your rough weight should be according to your height and build. From this you can work out how many calories a day you ought to be eating.

DESIRED WEIGHTS FOR MEN AND WOMEN
ACCORDING TO HEIGHT AND FRAME

MEN

HEIGHT IN FEET	SMALL FRAME	MEDIUM FRAME	LARGE FRAME
5' 02"	112-120	118-129	126-141
5' 03"	115-123	121-133	129-144
5'04"	118-126	124-136	132-148
5' 05"	121-129	127-139	135-152
5' 06"	124-133	130-143	138-156
5' 07"	128-137	134-147	142-161
5' 08"	132-141	138-152	147-166
5' 09"	136-145	142-156	151-170
5' 10"	140-150	146-160	155-174
5' 11"	144-154	150-165	159-179
6'	148-158	154-170	164-184
6' 01"	152-162	158-175	168-189
6'02"	156-167	162-180	173-194

NB Weight is given in pounds.

WOMEN

HEIGHT IN FEET	SMALL FRAME	MEDIUM FRAME	LARGE FRAME
4'10"	92-98	96-107	104-119
4' 11"	94-101	98-110	106-122
5'	96-104	101-113	109-125
5' 01"	96-104	101-113	109-125
5' 01"	99-107	104-116	112-128
5' 02"	102-110	107-119	115-131
5' 03"	105-113	110-122	118-134
5' 04"	108-116	113-126	121-138
5' 05"	111-119	116-130	125-142
5' 06"	114-123	120-135	129-146
5' 07"	118-127	124-139	133-150
5' 08"	122-131	128-143	137-154
5' 09"	126-135	132-147	141-148
5' 10"	130-140	136-151	145-163
5' 11"	134-144	140-155	149-168
6'	138-148	144-159	153-173

(Source: Build and Blood Pressure Study, Society of Actuaries.)

The chart shows the optimum weight a man and woman ought to be (rather than your actual weight). An adult man with a moderately active life style will require 15 calories per pound. Women have a slightly different metabolism. A moderate active woman burns fewer calories per pound. She needs 12 calories per pound. The calculations to work this out are as follows:

Imagine you are a women whose height is 5' 4' with a medium frame, weighing 160 pounds. According to the chart you should weigh not more than 126 pounds. Your calories intake should be calculated as follows:

126 X 12 = 1512 calories (moderately active woman)
126 X 10 = 1260 calories (inactive woman)
126 X 13 = 1638 calories. (with aerobic exercise)

Imagine you are a man whose height is 5' 7" with a medium frame weighing 180 pounds. According to the chart you should weigh no more than 147 pounds. Your calories intake should be calculated as follows:

147 X15 = 2205 calories (moderately active man)
147 X13 = 1911 calories (inactive man)
147 X16 = 2352 calories. (With exercise)

Eating Plan Summary

You may find it difficult to believe (if you've swallowed a library full of diet industry hype) but this chapter contains everything you need to know and use, to strip away just as much excess fat as your heart desires.

You know roughly what level of calorific content you should be aiming for, and how that content should be made up in terms of the proportion of carbohydrate, fat and protein. You also have a fairly comprehensive list of common foods with their nutritional content neatly summarised.

Armed with this information, you could put together, and then adhere to, the perfect eating plan – specifically tailored for you. But you won't do that of course, because you're human and you want a life!

But what I hope you will do, is use the information in this chapter to make some comfortable adjustments to the way you eat...adjustments you can stick to most of the time, and which over the long haul, will have a marked positive effect on your body.

It's small changes carried through over a long period of time, which make lasting changes to the way you look.

PROGRAMME SUMMARY

Wow! I've just re-read what I've written, and realised that I've gone in to far more detail on the background to the system than I intended. That's enthusiasm for you!

But the last thing I want to do, is give anyone the idea that this is complicated, because it isn't. By way of proof, I just want to summarise the rationale behind all this as succinctly as possible. If nothing else, it will act as an easy to access reminder of the core ideas and principles underpinning the system.

The Vince Graham System is about the way you look. It's not designed with fitness, general health or sports performance in mind (although it will help with all three). The goal of the programme is to get you in the best aesthetic shape possible, in the shortest possible time.

Muscles are what give shape to your body. In order to change your shape you have to impact on your muscles, and the only proven way to do that, is via some form of resistance training. Resistance training places unusual demands on the muscles, which (if it's done right) they respond to by getting bigger and stronger during rest.

Most resistance training programmes fail for a number of reasons...

1. People don't stick to the programme because it's too time consuming, inconvenient or boring.

2. The programme doesn't work the muscles intensely enough.

3. The programme lacks variety.

4. The programme doesn't allow adequate rest.

The best programmes fall down on one of these points...the worst fall down on all of them! The Vince Graham System addresses and attacks each of these potential downfalls...

- Vince's programme exercises the muscles for just 7 minutes a day, so time and boredom cease to become issues.

- The programme is extremely convenient. It can be done at home, and without any special equipment.

- Each session focuses on one muscle group, thereby facilitating the level of intensity required for progress.

- Workouts for individual muscle groups are on a four week cycle, thereby introducing the variety you need to keep subjecting the muscles to unusual demands.

- The programme places 7 days between individual muscle group workouts, thereby ensuring adequate recovery and rest.

It's this unique combination of convenience, intensity, focus, variety and rest...together with Vince's adaptation of some pretty advanced exercise principles, which create a very powerful synergy.

If your idea of the 'perfect body' is that of a professional bodybuilder, then this system isn't going to do it for you. You'll need to set aside at least 2 hours a day and a substantial pharmaceutical budget! If you want to look like a marathon runner, (though I can't imagine why you would) just get out and run...maybe the scrawny emaciated look will come back one day.

But if your goal is to sculpt the sort of body which you can be proud of...one which will be universally admired, (and envied)...then my final urging would be to put this book down now, and start putting Vince Graham's system to work for you.

Don't wait until New Year, or your birthday, or the end of the month, or the beginning of next week...or any other concocted starting date. At best, all that will do is delay you from reaching your goal. At worst it will stop you getting started altogether.

The hardest part of all is to begin, which is why I want you to do it now, while you're thinking about it. Every journey, whatever its length, starts with a single step. Make that step today.

Good luck, and keep me informed on your progress.